Naturopathy
Modern Way of Life

Published by :
Lotus Press Publishers & Distributors

Naturopathy
Modern Way of Life

Kishan Kumar Suman

Lotus
PRESS
4735/22, Prakash Deep Building
Ansari Road, Darya Ganj,
New Delhi - 110002

Lotus Press : Publishers & Distributors
Unit No. 220, 2nd Floor, 4735/22, Prakash Deep Building,
Ansari Road, Darya Ganj, New Delhi- 110002
Ph.: 41325510, 98118-38000
• E-mail : lotuspress1984@gmail.com
www.lotuspress.co.in

Naturopathy Modern Way of Life

ISBN: 978-81-8382-225-1

Printed & Published by : **Lotus Press Publishers & Distributors,** New Delhi-02

Preface

Naturopathy (also known as naturopathic medicine or natural medicine) is an eclectic alternative medical system that focuses on natural remedies, and the body's vital ability to heal and maintain itself. It is a distinct, integrated system of primary health care offered by licensed physicians.

It consists of the diagnosis, treatment, and prevention of human disorders by the therapeutic use of natural methods and materials. These might include Clinical Nutrition, Herbal Medicine, Hygiene, Homeoopathy, Naturopathic Manipulation, or ancient medical systems like those of China or India.

There is a wide range of conditions that naturopathic doctors treat, either alone or in combination with other complementary or usual medical treatments. These include acute conditions such as headaches, sore throats, ear infections, intestinal upsets, colds and flu, etc.; chronic illnesses such as migraines, musculoskeletal pain, gastrointestinal, gynecological, arthritis, heart disease, etc.; inherent tendencies before they become a serious illness or degenerative disease; mental and emotional problems to reduce the effects of recent stresses and long-term patterns of anger, depression or anxiety; and physical injury and trauma, including possible referral to appropriate specialists.

Naturopathic philosophy favours a holistic approach and minimal use of surgery and drugs. Naturopathy comprises many different treatment modalities of varying degrees of acceptance by the medical community; diet and lifestyle advice may be substantially similar to that offered by non-naturopaths, and acupuncture may help reduce pain in some cases, but homoeopathy is often characterised as pseudoscience.

Naturopathy is built upon the dictum of Hippocrates, the father of medicine, who declared "Nature cures; not the physicians." Hippocrates and his colleagues considered disease to be an effect of some imbalance in the elements like air, water and other natural factors such as food.

Naturopathy is primarily and fundamentally drugless and bloodless, yet in its broader aspects it does admit the use of both natural medicine and surgery when their use is constructive. The techniques employed in nature cure vary with the experience of its practitioner.

Someone had once remarked that there would come a time when there is likely to be a reverse migration to the countryside. Perhaps mindsets are beginning to change already, and 'return to nature' is the mantra of the new millennium. Indeed, it is in nature that mankind is likely to find solutions to its myriad problems, health-related or otherwise.

Author

Content

1
Introduction

What is Naturopathy?

Naturopathy is the system of healiNaturopathy Modern Way of Lifeng in which diseases are cured by means of all natural and rational remedies such as light, water, air, heat, exercise, diet and other physiological measures. It is a combination of different methods of natural healing.

It is a system of non-invasive health care and health assessment, in which neither surgery nor drugs are used; dependence being placed only on education, counselling, naturopathic modalities and natural substances, including the use of foods, food extracts, vitamins, minerls, enzymes, digestive aids, botanical substances, topical natural substances, homoeopathic preparations, air, water, heat, cold, sound, light; the physical modalities of magnetic therapy, naturopathic non-manipulative body work and exercise to help stimulate and maintain the individual's intrinsic self-healing processes.

Naturopathic medicine is a distinct healing philosophy and practice, which seeks to promote health, by using the body's life-force and inner protecting mechanism for stimulating and supporting the body's inherent power of regaining harmony and balance.

Naturopathy believes that all forms of disease are due to the same cause, that is, the accumulation of waste materials and toxins in our bodies that are steadily piling up. Fasting to relieve the symptoms of an upset stomach, using water as a healing aid or eating a sensible balanced diet to maintain good health are all examples of naturopathy.

It is also a way of life. In fact, Nature Cure is a way of life of which we find a number of references in the *Vedas* and other ancient texts. The morbid matter theory, concept of vital force and other concepts upon which Nature Cure is based are already available in old texts which indicate that these methods were widely practised in ancient India. It is known by different names: Nature Cure, the natural methods, the New Science of Healing and Healing from Within.

It is an important aspect of Naturopathy.

Origin of Naturopathy

The origins of the practice can be traced back over two thousand years to the time of Hippocrates. The basis of the modern practice can be traced back to the beginning of the 19th century and to people such as Preissnitz, a therapist in Germany, who used the beneficial effects of water as a therapy (hydrotherapy).

Towards the end of the 19th century in Bavaria, Father Kneipp, a monk, who was obviously a naturopath, treated an American Benedictine by the name of Lust. As a result of his recovery, Lust stayed with Kneipp to study his particular methods of healing, and upon returning to the United States he established his own form of natural medicine which he called naturopathy. The blend of therapies employed by him included nutrition and natural diet, homoeopathy, herbal medicine, hydrotherapy, chiropractic and the management of stress.

Thus at the beginning of the 19th century, Naturopathy began to be formally recognised. The term 'Naturopathy' was created by Dr. Scheel of New York city.

Focus of Naturopathy

We live in a largely synthetic and artificial world. A world that has increasingly stepped away from nature. This denial of the pristine, has contributed to many of the ills that plague modern living. Naturopathy or cure through Nature is as old as life on earth. Animals have used the bounty of Mother Nature for aeons, for every ailment ever encountered by them.

Ever since our advent on planet earth, we have not only used the cures offered by nature, but with typical human ingenuity, have created diverse applications and usages of herbs, medicinal plants, leaves, barks, roots.

Entire systems of medicine have grown around the curative processes of extracts from plants.

Entire cultures, from the Druids of the West to Medicine Men of Africa, to the Vaids of India, have discovered, sustained, enhanced and preserved the curative power of Nature in different, but complementary ways.

There are two areas of focus in naturopathy: one is supporting the body's own healing abilities, and the other is empowering individuals to make lifestyle changes necessary for the best possible health. While naturopathic doctors treat both short bouts of illness and chronic conditions, their emphasis is on prevention of disease and patient education.

Naturopathy advocates a new lifestyle with corrective habits, such as exercise, a good diet and a moderate approach towards all things. In naturopathy, the fundamental healing force is considered to be nature itself, that is, the power of the individual to defeat disease. Nature cure attempts to invigorate the system, to build up blood and lymph, and to purify the tissues so that germ activity is rendered inconsequential.

An unhealthy lifestyle can cause many diseases. So it is

better to avoid a diet high in fat, salt and refined carbohydrates, smoking, excess consumption of alcohol and high stress levels. Naturopathic lifestyle should be viewed as a method of disease prevention.

Nature cure believes that disease is one, its cause is one and so its treatment is one.

Naturopathy: A Holistic System of Treatment

A 'holistic' system of medicine or healing has become the buzzword in recent times. Thus, naturopathy, homoeopathy, magneto therapy, acupressure, acupuncture, ayurveda, the unani system of medicine, etc., have been gaining in popularity. In treating patients, the naturopathic practitioner may use a number of alternative therapies, including homoeopathy, herbal remedies, traditional Chinese medicine, spinal manipulation, nutrition, hydrotherapy, massage and exercise.

The whole approach of these systems of medicine differs from allopathy inasmuch as that the ingredients of remedies are not chemicals, artificially produced in laboratories. They are natural substances like extracts from plants, animals or minerals. They have no side effects, are gentle on the human system and aim at reviving the organism into expelling toxins and getting rid of diseases by rejuvenating the body's own defence mechanism.

Even systems like acupressure and acupuncture focus on the 'Vita flex' points on the palms and feet. By applying selective pressure or puncturing nodal prints with extremely thin needles the body's own defence mechanism is activated into fighting disease, and organs associated with the corresponding points are strengthened.

Even aromatherapy has been gaining in popularity in recent times. It is the system in which the aroma of herbs and flowers is inhaled for curative purposes. The oil obtained from flowers is even massaged on the

Vita Flex points on the feet and other strategic locations of the body.

How do Waste Materials pile up?

Nature Cure believes that all the diseases arise due to accumulation of morbid matter in the body, and if scope is given for its removal, it provides cure or relief. It also believes that the human body possesses inherent self- constructing and self-healing powers. The fundamental difference in Nature Cure with other systems is that its theory and practice are based on holistic viewpoint whereas the latter's approach is specific. Nature Cure does not believe in the specific cause of disease and its specific treatment but takes into account the totality of factors responsible for diseases such as one's unnatural habits in living, thinking, working, sleeping, relaxation, sexual indulgence etc, and also considers the environmental factors involved which on the whole disturbs the normal functioning of the body and lead it to a morbid, weak and toxic state.

***Natural means* :** Our body is made up of cells, some of which continuously die and are replaced by new ones. The old dead cells are foreign material to the body and need to be eliminated. In addition, processes of the living cells also generate toxic wastes due to metabolic reactions.

***Unnatural means*:** Wrong ways of life also cause production of excess toxins. When these toxins are not eliminated at a reasonably fast rate, a diseased condition is created

Germs do not cause disease but are found breeding in the accumulating waste matter in the body. In a healthy body, having normal secretions and excretions, the germs cannot find a breeding ground and are destroyed by the antibodies present in the secretions. There have been extensive experiments to prove this.

"Just as mud cannot stick to a smooth, oily surface, similarly, the germs cannot blemish a healthy body."

Germs are part of the result of disease and not the cause.

Nature Cure recognises this. Instead of concentrating its energy on killing germs, the activity of which we cannot escape when the conditions are ripe.

The whole practice of Nature cure based on the following three principles:

1. Accumulation of morbid matter
2. Abnormal composition of blood and lymph
3. Lowered vitality

Importance of Exercise, Yoga and a Conducive Lifestyle

Exercise keeps the balance between nutrition and drainage. Exercise, both physical and mental, help greatly in removing toxins. Exercises provide for a greater intake of oxygen and help in improving blood circulation. Organ massage also takes place. Yoga provides for an extremely bene-ficial and complete method aimed at total body and mind health.

People seek naturopathic care for various health-related purposes, including primary care, support of wellness, and treatment of diseases and conditions (often chronic ones). Naturopathy helps to prevent many common diseases such as headaches, common cold, hypertension, peptic ulcers and many of the disorders associated with ageing, including diabetes. It aims at educating people about adopting the type of lifestyle which is conducive to good health.

The Healing Power of Nature

The foundation of naturopathic medicine is the philosophy of the healing power of nature. This means that within every human organism there is a healing energy, which influences our immune system in the fuller sense of both the physical and the psychic.

Following this first premise is the second, that the therapies used to support and stimulate this healing power of nature must be in "the gentlest, least invasive, most efficient manner possible".

The third naturopathic premise is "to diagnose and treat the cause". Naturopaths do not simply treat the manifestation of the disease, but seek the cause and treat it.

Naturopathic medicine is a holistic approach to health. Disease affects the mind and spirit as well, not simply an isolated organ or system. Each person responds in a unique way to his or her physical environment; each has individual vitality and strength.

Each person has different inherited tendencies and genetic patterns. While treating the whole person, the naturopathic practitioner searches for causes at many levels and attempts to eliminate the fundamental cause of illness, and not simply to relieve symptoms.

The earliest doctors and healers worked with herbs, foods, water, fasting and tissue manipulation — gentle treatments that do not obscure the body's own healing powers. Today's naturopathic physicians continue to use these therapies as their main tools and to advocate a healthy dose of primary prevention. In addition, modern naturopaths conduct and make practical use of the latest biochemical research involving nutrition, botanicals, homoeopathy, and other natural treatments.

A central belief in naturopathy is that nature has a healing power (a principle called *vis medicatrix naturae*). Another belief is that living organisms (including the human body) have the power to maintain (or return to) a state of balance and health, and to heal themselves. Practitioners of naturopathy prefer to use treatment approaches that they consider to be the most natural and least invasive, instead of using drugs and more invasive procedures.

For many diseases and conditions (a few examples are ulcerative colitis, asthma, menopause, flu, obesity and chronic fatigue), treatments used by naturopathic physicians can be primary and even curative.

Naturopathic physicians also function within an integrated framework, for example referring patients to an appropriate medical specialist such as an oncologist or a surgeon. Naturopathic therapies can be employed within that context to complement the treatments used by conventionally trained medical doctors. The result is a team-care approach that recognises the needs of the patient to receive the best overall treatment most appropriate to his or her specific medical condition.

Criticisms

There are criticisms about the efficacy of naturapathy. Naturopathy is viewed with scepticism for its reliance on or association with unproven, disproven, and controversial alternative medical treatments, and for its vitalistic underpinnings. As with any alternative care, there is a risk of misdiagnosis; this risk may be lower depending on level of training. There is also a risk that ailments that cannot be diagnosed by naturopaths will go untreated while a patient attempts treatment programs designed by their naturopath. Certain naturopathic treatments, such as homeopathy and iridology, are widely considered pseudoscience or quackery.

Natural methods and chemicals are not necessarily safer or more effective than artificial or synthetic ones; any treatment capable of eliciting an effect may also have deleterious side effects.

Health Shops

Other than the regular homoeopaths, naturopaths and ayurveds, there are health shops now, that stock an exclusive range of health foods, like the one at Koregaon Park in Pune aptly titled, 'Natures Bounty', for instance. The shop sells health foods, organic cereals, low fat anytime snacks, natural vitamins and supplements, herbal cosmetics etc. Shops like that have on offer herbal dietary supplements to meet all kinds of health challenges, such as failing memory, a weak heart, obesity, water retention, weak liver, low energy, weak digestion, cardiovascular challenges, respiratory disorders, diabetes, low immunity, hormone balance, enlarged prostate etc.

That is not all, there are on offer these days, preparations for weight gain and loss and detoxifying agents to flush out all body toxins. They sell herbal 'Antibiotics' as well as 'Aphrodisiacs'. Beauty products for skin and hair care and increasing the size of breasts are also on offer. Moreover, mood creators – oils for concentration, increase of libido etc. —are also available. Lastly, products that are natural pesticides have gained in popularity in homes with kids.

Naturopathic Practitioners

K. C. Atwood writes in the journal *Medscape General Medicine*, "Naturopathic physicians now claim to be primary care physicians proficient in the practice of both conventional and natural medicine. Their training, however, amounts to a small fraction of that of medical doctors who practice primary care. An examination of their literature, moreover, reveals that it is replete with pseudoscientific, ineffective, unethical and potentially dangerous practices."

In the United States and Canada, the designation of Naturopathic Doctor (ND) may be awarded after a completion of a four-year programme of study at an accredited naturopathic medical school that includes the study of basic medical sciences as well as natural remedies and medical care.

In India, doctors of naturopathy train at accredited four-year naturopathy medical schools. The first two years include many of the same core science classes as regular medical schools, while the final two years focus on training in natural healing techniques. Here, there are two types of degrees awarded to the students, undergoing courses in naturopathy. The first are graduates of All India Naturopathy Council and are awarded DNYS (Diploma in Naturopathy and Yogic Sciences) after three years of guided study and internship. The second is the university graduates who are awarded BNYS (Bachelor of Naturopathy and Yogic Sciences). BNYS is a four-and-a-half-year course with one-year internship. The BNYS course is offered by several universities in India.

Traditional naturopaths are guided by the same naturopathic philosophies and principles as board-licensed naturopathic doctors and often prescribe similar treatments. Compared to naturopathic medical schools, traditional naturopaths' training programmes are less rigorous and do not provide the same basic and clinical science education.

A naturopathy doctor, or ND, may pay considerable attention to a patient's lifestyle, since naturopathy theory holds that physical, psychological and even spiritual elements can all contribute to disease.

Naturopathic medicine is usually practised by licensed physicians who have been trained by accredited schools. Every aspect of a disease or a disorder, including diagnoses, treatment and prevention, can be treated by naturopathic doctors. Naturopathic doctors may use herbal medicine, clinical nutrition, homoeopathy, naturopathic manipulation and Eastern philosophies to formulate a proper course of treatment.

One of the main goals of naturopathic doctors is to identify the underlying cause of an illness. They may examine physical, genetic, emotional and dietary factors that may have contributed to patient's present state. With natural remedies, they may suggest modifications to a patient's exercise regime and dietary habits and may advocate lifestyle changes.

Despite an emphasis on natural treatment, doctors who practise naturopathy may use some of the same tools that medical doctors use to treat patients. Blood tests and medical imaging can help naturopaths determine the exact cause of a disease, for instance. Minor surgery may even be performed on a patient. However, minor surgery, intravenous therapy and natural childbirth are areas that need to be further studied by the naturopath before he or she can perform them on patients.

2
History

The word "naturopathy" was first used in the US exactly 100 years ago. But the natural therapies and the philosophy on which naturopathy is based have been effectively used to treat diseases since ancient times.

As Rene Dubos noted in *The Mirage of Health* (1959), the word "physician" is from the Greek root meaning "nature".

Hippocrates, a physician who lived 2400 years ago, is often considered the earliest predecessor of naturopathic physicians, particularly in terms of his teaching that "nature is healer of all diseases" and his formulation of the concept *vis medicatrix naturae* — "the healing power of nature." This concept has long been at the core of indigenous medicine in many cultures around the world and remains one of the central themes of naturopathic philosophy to this day.

The word *naturopathy* comes from Greek and Latin and literally translates as "nature disease". The history of naturopathy could be traced back to 400 BC. It was practised in ancient Greece.

However, the modern form of naturopathy can be traced to 18th- and 19th-century natural healing systems. Such systems include hydrotherapy (water therapy), which was popular in Germany and nature cure, developed in Austria, and based on the use of food, air, light, water and herbs to treat illness.

Pioneers Kneipp and Lust

Dr. Benedict Lust, a German immigrant, is considered the founder of modern-day naturopathy. When Lust became seriously ill with what he believed was tuberculosis, he was treated by a priest and healer in Germany named Sebastian Kneipp. Kneipp's treatment was based on various healing approaches and philosophies that were popular in Europe, including hydrotherapy (water treatments). The "nature cure" movement focused on restoring health through a return to nature. This movement advocated therapies such as gentle exercise, herbal medications, wholesome dietary approaches, and exposure to sun and air. Lust found his health much improved from Kneipp's treatment, and when he immigrated to the United States at the turn of the 20th century, he was dedicated to popularising it. He gave it the name 'Naturopathy', and led the way in the United States.

Dr. Lust not only practised the art of natural healing but also introduced it in the US in the year 1892, developing it as a medical system. In 1902, he established the American School of Naturopathy.

The years 1902 to 1917 were the formative period of naturopathic medicine and art of natural healing in the US. Dr. Lust stressed on the hygiene, diet habits, hydrotherapy and emotional strength as essential tools for a healthy body. He merged herbalism with naturopathic healing.

The years 1918 to 1937 were known as the halcyon years. During this period, naturopathy gained importance, and the general public not only supported but also showed a keen interest in naturopathic medicines and therapies. Many states in the US introduced naturopathic licensure laws during these halcyon years.

In the mid-1920s to 1940, while allopathic medical training and pharmaceuticals, and medical technologies gained notoriety, the use of naturopathic medicine declined. Many naturopathic journals were circulated among the general public in the US. This was done to provide information on how to prevent disease and maintain a healthy lifestyle. Naturopathic journals emphasized on the eating habits of the common man and focused on taking measures to correct poor eating habits. Naturopathy advice is to include fibre-rich food, and its stress is on cutting down on red meat.

In 1945, Dr. Benedict Lust died. After his death, there was a decline in usage of naturopathic medicines and therapies. During this period more importance was given to allopathic medicines and treatment.

Rejuvenation of Naturopathy

In the 1960s, the general public became more aware of the good nutrition and healthy lifestyles. During this period importance was given to alternative medicines and naturopathy was rejuvenated.

In 1978, the first naturopathic college, known as the National College of Naturopathic Medicine, was established in America. This was the first legitimate college for naturopathy.

In 1987, Bastyr University became the first naturopathic college to be accredited and recognised by the Council on Naturopathic Medical (CAM) Education. Today it is part of complementary and alternative medicine, a group of diverse medical and health care systems, practices, and products that are not presently considered to be part of conventional medicine. Complementary medicine is used together with conventional medicine, and alternative medicine is used in place of conventional medicine.

Today, naturopathy is practised widely not only in the US but around the globe. It was not until the 1960s that naturopathic-style holistic medicine regained popularity. Today, naturopaths are licensed care providers in many states offering information and a variety of alternative and complementary therapies, including homoeopathy, vitamin and mineral supplements, traditional Chinese medicine, relaxation techniques, and herbal remedies.

Naturopathy in India

In India, the Government of India, after having recognised the need for systematic research and development of yoga and naturopathy in the country, established the Central Council for Research in Ayurveda, Yoga & Naturopathy (CCRYN), Unani, Siddha and Homoeopathy in 1969 as an autonomous organisation under the Ministry of Health and Family Welfare. This organisation, the first of its kind, was established in India by the Central Government to conduct scientific research in ayurveda, siddha, unani and yoga, and it existed up to 1978. During this period, the development of naturopathy was looked after by the Ministry of Health & Family Welfare directly. Later, in March 1978, this composite Council (CCRYN) was dissolved to pave way for the formation of four independent Research Councils, one each for ayurveda and siddha, unani, homoeopathy, yoga and naturopathy. Hence, this Council (CCRYN) was established in 1978 with a view to provide better opportunities for all-round development of yoga and naturopathy independently according to their own doctrines and fundamental principles.

The National Institute of Naturopathy, Pune, came into existence on 22 December 1986. It encourages facilities for standardisation and propagation of the existing knowledge and its application through research in naturopathy throughout India. This Institute has a Governing Body headed by Union Minister for Health as its President.

In India the Nature Cure movement gained momentum during the times of Mahatma Gandhi. As the 'Father of the Nation' became interested in this system and realised its benefits, he made it a part of his programmes. The influence of naturopathy on him is fortified by the fact that he even established a Nature Cure Hospital in Uruli Kanchan, District Poona, Maharashtra, which is still functional. Since then, numerous naturopathic hospitals have opened up in the country. However, it should be noted that the Indian stream of naturopathy differs from the Western stream in many ways, particularly in their emphasis on strict vegetarianism and yoga.

Naturopathy is very popular in India, and there are numerous naturopathy hospitals in the country. There are also many doctors trained in the Western system of medicine who have acquired naturopathy degrees so as to integrate the insights gained into their system of practice.

Most of the principles and practices of naturopathy like Morbid Matter Theory, Fasting, Nutrition, Dietetics, Cleansing acts, Exercises, Massage, Longevity have been in practice in some form or another, and are well known to our ancient vaidyas, seers and saints. Because of this, natural modalities and concepts form an integral part of Indian way of living, thinking tradition and culture.

Today, naturopathy is quickly growing in popularity and accepted use

The system grew in popularity towards the close of the 1900s, and today there are two streams of naturopaths in India. The first are graduates of All India Naturopathy Council and are awarded DNYS (Diploma in Naturopathy and Yogic Sciences) after three years of guided study and internship. The second are university graduates who are awarded BNYS (Bachelor of Naturopathy and Yogic Sciences).

BNYS is a four and half year course with a one-year internship. The BNYS course is offered by S. D. M. College of Naturopathy and Yogic Sciences, which is the first college in India to offer a five-year degree course in Naturopathy and Yogic Sciences. The college was first part of the University of Mangalore from 1989 to 2000, but later was shifted to the Rajiv Gandhi University of Health Science, Bangalore, after the formation of a health university.

Another college that offers degree courses is the Government Gandhi Nature Cure College, Hyderabad, India, which is affiliated with NTR University of Health Sciences, J.S.S. Institute of Naturopathy and Yogic Sciences, under T.N.M.G.R. Medical University. A lot of colleges have since been developed in India.

Rishikesh in India is called the yoga capital of the world and there are many ashrams in Rishikesh offering courses on meditation, yoga and Hindu philosophy. The International Yoga Festival is organised every year from February 2 to 7 by the state tourism. Kerala, in the southernmost tip of India, is noted, among many other things, for its ayurvedic resorts that draw a large number of tourists every year.

The treatments provided by these resorts have become so popular that the Kerala Tourism Development Corporation has started a 'Monsoon Rejuvenation' Package that combines sightseeing tours with ayurvedic massages and treatment. The ayurvedic treatments are considered most effective after the monsoon months because during this period the body has less heat and hence is most responsive to treatments.

Naturopathic treatments are given in different places in India. Recently, naturopathy is widely used and become popular at international level because it is an effective and protected healing, technique. Since natural herbs are used for healing therefore no side effects are visible. India is using old tradition of ayurveda and yoga, so it has become a naturopathy hub. In today's busy schedule and heavy workload give birth to numerous physical disorder and mental stress, anxiety, which may increase blood sugar levels, pressure and cholesterol.

3

Principles of Naturopathy

Naturopathy is a healing method that has its roots in almost all the cultures. India's ayurveda, traditional Chinese and Greek medicine, all lay great emphasis on the natural healing system. They believe that the body has natural abilities to resist diseases and to heal itself. Naturopathic medicine is a natural approach to health and healing that recognises the integrity of the whole person.

Naturopathic medicine represents the vitalistic tradition of medicine in today's world. That is, it treats a disease through the stimulation, increase and support of the person's inherent healing capacity. These treatments are chosen to work with the patient's vital force, respecting the natural healing processes of nature.

Principles of Healing

The practice of naturopathic medicine includes six underlying principles of healing. These are based on the observation of health and disease. This observation process involves the use of modern scientific methodologies and language. The following principles make naturopathic medicine different from all other medical approaches:

1. Do no harm.

Illness is a purposeful process of the organism. The process of healing includes the generation of symptoms which are, in fact, an expression of the life force-attempting to heal itself.

Therapeutic actions should be complementary to and synergistic with this healing process.

Utilise methods and medical substances which minimise the risk of harmful side effects, using the least force necessary to diagnose and treat.

Avoid when possible the harmful suppression of symptoms.

Acknowledge, respect and work with the individual's self-healing process.

Refer for appropriate treatment when naturopathic therapies are inappropriate. The physician's actions can support or antagonise the actions of the healing power of Nature. Therefore, methods designed to suppress symptoms without removing the underlying causes are considered harmful and to be avoided or minimised.

2. The healing power of Nature.

The body has an inherent ability to establish, maintain and restore health. The healing process is ordered and intelligent; nature heals through the response of the life force.

The physician's role is to facilitate this process, to identify and remove obstacles to health and recovery, and to establish or restore a healthy internal and external environment.

3. Identify and treat the cause.

The root cause of all diseases is supposed to be the accumulation of foreign matter and waste products in the body. In a diseased state the body excretes all foreign matter and waste products. Naturopathy hence tries to eliminate the root cause of illness. It does not suppress symptoms because it might interfere with healing.

Illness does not occur without cause. Underlying causes of disease must be discovered and removed or treated before a person can recover completely from illness.

Symptoms express the body's attempt to heal, but are not the cause of disease. Symptoms, therefore, should not be suppressed by treatment.

Causes may occur on many levels including physical, mental, emotional and spiritual. The physician must evaluate fundamental underlying causes on all levels, directing treatment at root causes rather than at symptomatic expression.

4. Heal the whole person.

Health and disease are conditions of the whole organism, a whole involving the complex interaction of many factors. The naturopathic physician must treat the whole person by taking these factors into account. The harmonious functioning of physical, mental, emotional and spiritual aspects are essential to recovery from and prevention of disease. This requires a comprehensive approach to diagnosis and treatment.

5. The physician as teacher.

A cooperative doctor-patient relationship has inherent therapeutic value. The physician's major role is to educate and encourage the patient to take responsibility for his own health. The physician is a catalyst for healthful change, empowering and motivating the patient to assume responsibility. It is the patient, not the doctor, who ultimately creates/accomplishes healing. Teaching with hope, knowledge and understanding, the physician acts to enable patients to heal.

6. Prevention is the best cure.

The ultimate goal of any health care system should be prevention of disease. This is accomplished through education and promotion of life-habits that create good health. The physician learns to assess risk factors and to sharpen their deductive reasoning, and understand the patient's circumstances. Appropriate interventions are then sought to avoid further harm or risk to the patient. Building health works better and more surely than fighting disease.

In short, Nature Cure includes all the available non-invasive treatments and diagnostic modalities which do not interfere with the body's natural functional capacity and healing process and are in infirmity with Nature's constructive principles.

Naturopathy is a system of healing science stimulating the body's inherent power to regain health with the help of five great elements of nature – Earth, Water, Air, Fire and Ether. Naturopathy is a call to "Return to Nature" and to resort to simple way of living in harmony with the self, society and environment.

Naturopathy provides not only a simple practical approach to the management of diseases, but a firm theoretical basis which is applicable to all the holistic medical care and by giving attention to the foundations of health; also offers a more economical frame work for the medicine of future generation.

Prana is the vitality force. Naturopathy aims at providing life force to the body by protecting it from internal and external threats. It helps in physical and mental well being. This can be achieved by harmonious and coordinated functioning of the five elements of nature.

Control over senses is the foundation of good health. A well planned life and positive thinking has a favourable effect on the healing process. Simple or *sattvic* food, proper rest, sound sleep, cleanliness and peaceful mind are the features of a planned life-style.

Naturopathy believes that every body has germs that grow and multiply. To prevent germ growth, it prescribes to clean and purify the body regularly.

The techniques applicable to naturopathic treatment of disease and illness are the same techniques applicable to treatment by an allopath, with greater emphasis upon hydrotherapy, massage, manipulation, or electrotherapy in necessary instances, and with greater utilization of medications in their natural or botanical form than in their chemically-created or derived form.

Nature cure physicians do not believe in giving poisonous drugs to kill germs. They rather purify the blood and tissues to develop immunity. Lowered vitality and increase of toxic and morbid matter in the body causes a diseased state. Increase in cholesterol leads to high blood pressure and risk of heart attack.

The naturopathic approach to health care can prevent minor illnesses from developing into more serious or chronic degenerative diseases. Patients are taught the principles for living a healthy life. By following these principles, they are more likely to prevent major illnesses and promote health and well-being.

To sum up:

1. All diseases, their causes and their treatments are one.
2. The basic cause of disease is not bacteria. Bacteria develop after the accumulation of morbid matter when a favourable atmosphere for their growth develops in the body. The basic cause is morbid matter and not the bacteria.
3. Acute diseases are our friends, not the enemies. Chronic diseases are the outcome of wrong treatment and suppression of the acute diseases.
4. Nature is the greatest healer. The body has the capacity to prevent itself from diseases and regain health if unhealthy.
5. In naturopathy the patient is treated and not the disease.
6. In naturopathy the diagnosis is easily possible. Ostentation is not required. Long waiting for the diagnosis is not required for the treatment.
7. Patients suffering from chronic ailments are also treated successfully in comparatively less time in naturopathy.
8. After emerging, suppressed diseases can be cured by naturopathy.
9. Nature Cure treats physical, mental, social (moral) and spiritual, all four aspects at the same time.

10. Nature Cure treats body as a whole instead of giving treatment to each organ separately.
11. Naturopathy does not use medicines. According to Naturopathy "Food is Medicine".

In short, Nature Cure includes all the available non-invasive treatments and diagnostic modalities which do not interefere with the body's natural functional capacity and healing process, and are in harmony with Nature's constructive principles.

4

Practice and Methods

Naturopathy treatment is a practice of treating diseases by prescribing natural medicines. It is a form of treatment which emphasizes the tendency of the body to retain a sense of balance and cure itself. Naturopathy treatments are non toxic and stimulate healing and cleansing responses in a patient.

Naturopathy involves diagnosis and prescription of modalities and methods of nature. Naturopathic medicines mainly include water, earth, air, light, heat and diet therapy.

Naturopathic doctors (ND) treat the whole person, which means they consider a variety of factors before they diagnose and treat an illness. Factors an ND might consider in making a diagnosis include your mental, emotional, and spiritual state, your diet, your family history (whether or not your parents or grandparents suffer (or suffered) from the same condition), your environment, and your lifestyle.

Some of the more common treatments used by a naturopath include:

1. Nutritional Counselling

Your intern or naturopathic doctor may ask you to keep a diet diary, which is the first step in helping to determine:

1. Food allergies
2. Sensitivities
3. Digestive issues
4. Risk for disease associated with diet, and

5. Overall diet quality

Clinicians can then recommend dietary changes to support healthy living and treat diseases like:

1. Diabetes
2. High cholesterol, and
3. Heart disease

2. Herbal Medicine

This therapy uses medications prepared by plants and plant extracts. Colonic irrigation or colon hydrotherapy: this form of therapy involves the use of medicinal remedies mixed with water to detoxify the body.

Herbal or botanical medicine has been used for thousands of years. Today, 80 per cent of the world's population uses plants to treat illness. Many conventional drugs used today were originally derived from medicinal plants. Plants are used medicinally because they do not have high toxicity, accumulate in the body, or cause habituation or withdrawal symptoms.

Herbs are used to enhance immune function; improve digestion; normalise bodily functions; destroy bacteria, viruses, and fungi; soothe irritated tissues; calm nerves and relax muscles. Even though scientific studies are validating the use of many herbs, herbal practitioners still prescribe herbs based on empirical evidence and tradition.

Herbs can be taken in many forms:

1. Herbal tea
2. Compress (fomentation)
3. Poultice
4. Tincture
5. Syrup
6. Gargle
7. Douche
8. Bath

9. Salve
10. Suppositories

3. Homoeopathic Medicine

It is a therapy in which the sick are given minute doses of remedy that would produce the symptoms of the disease in a healthy person.

Homoeopathic medicines or "remedies" use minute amounts of plant, mineral or animal substances to stimulate a person's innate healing ability and to strengthen the entire system. It attempts to treat "like with like", using substances that, in larger dosages, would develop the illness's symptom in a healthy person. The causes of your symptoms are unique to you; therefore, your intern or ND will examine the cause of your pain or illness before prescribing appropriate homoeopathic remedies.

Homoeopathy restores the body to homeostasis, or healthy balance, which is considered its natural state. The symptoms of a disease are regarded as the body's own defensive attempt to correct its imbalance, rather than as enemies to be defeated. Homoeopathic remedies are designed to stimulate this internal curative process rather than suppress the symptoms.

Homoeopathic remedies are particularly effective for:

1. Depression
2. Anxiety
3. Allergies
4. Infections
5. Gynecological concerns
6. Skin conditions
7. Digestive problems
8. Chronic and acute conditions including colds and flu
   Homeopathy is a popular therapy throughout the world, particularly in Great Britain, Europe and India. It is also gaining popularity with veterinarians, who offer homoeopathic remedies to treat dogs, cats and other animals.

4. Acupuncture

It is a method of inserting and controlling filiform needles into specific body points for therapeutic purpose and to heal pain.

5. Acupressure

There are different points on hands, feet & body which are associated with different organs. By applying pressure on these selected points, related organs can be influenced for getting rid of their ailments.

6. Hydrotherapy (water therapy)

Therapies in this category include drinking natural spring water, taking baths, alternating hot and cold applications, and exercising in water, all of which are thought to stimulate and support healing and strengthen the immune system.

7. Physical Medicine

This natural approach to healing involves using touch, hot and cold compresses, electric currents, and sound waves to manipulate the muscles, bones, and spine.

Physical medicine includes massage, hydrotherapy, peat therapy and other physical therapies such as ultraviolet and infrared therapy. Physical medicine works in two ways. First, it restores structural soundness to the skeletal system, joints and soft tissue. In addition, it builds immunity and supports healing and detoxification.

Many ways are offered by naturopaths to improve your well-being, recover from your injuries and strengthen your immune system. You may be referred to our pain management and sports medicine clinic for certain health concerns, such as:

1. Chronic pain
2. Arthritis
3. Sports injuries, and
4. Muscle strains

Treatments offered include:

1. Various massage techniques
2. Muscle-stretching, and
3. Manipulation of the spine and extremities

8. Detoxification

This therapy removes toxins from the body by using techniques such as fasting, enemas, and drinking water in large amounts.

9. Spirituality

Personal spiritual development is encouraged as an important part of an overall health program.

10. Lifestyle and Psychological Counselling

An ND may use hypnosis, guided imagery, or other counselling methods as part of a treatment plan.

To achieve the best results from your naturopathic treatment, you need to understand and practise the principles of healthy living. By helping you identify and adjust the habits that contribute to ill health, your intern or naturopath will help you maintain wellness over the long term.

Mental attitudes and emotions are important elements in overall health and should be considered when treating illness and disease. As part of their education, naturopathic doctors are trained in various counselling techniques. Lifestyle counselling, in conjunction with other naturopathic therapies, can provide support for those dealing with depression, fatigue, seasonal affective disorder (SAD), work-related stress, relationship issues, life transitions, and health problems, particularly chronic health problems.

11. Abstinence

This form of therapy includes voluntarily restraining certain appetites and desires that give pleasure. It also takes in discontinuing an addictive drug

12. Diet

A suitable diet is prescribed and regular check is kept on the diet of an individual. Most of the disease are amenable through food therapy. As you eat so will you be physically as well as mentally. Your food is your medicine. These are the main slogans of Nature Cure.

13. Fasting

It was first promoted by rishis and gurus in India. Fasting is an excellent treatment for obesity, arthritis, high blood pressure, cold, rheumatism, sinusitis and allergies. Fasting provides the body mechanisms to rest and rejuvenate.

14. Mud Treatment

Mud is applied to the skin and enclosed in a thin cotton wrapper. Mudpacks are very helpful in removing toxins from the body. Mud absorbs, dissolves and eliminates the toxins and rejuvenates the body. It is employed in treatment of various diseases like constipation, skin diseases etc.

15. Massage

Massage is generally employed for tonic, stimulant and sedative effects. It is an effective substitute for exercise. Massages tone muscles and give them strength. They also improve blood circulation.

16. Sunbath

Sunshine helps the body to produce vitamin D

17. Exercise and Yoga

Yoga and exercise keeps you fit and healthy. It improves blood circulation and tones muscles. It helps in loosing body weight.

18. Relaxation

The cause for most of the diseases is lack of proper physical and mental rest. Techniques like Shavasana and Yoganindra are prescribed for proper rest and relaxation.

19. Zone Reflexology

Commonly known as Acupressure, this therapy rejuvenates the nervous system. It also improves and balances the working of various organs and glands.

20. Magnet Therapy

Magnets influence health. South and North poles of different powers and shapes are employed in treatment, by applying directly on different parts of the body or through charged up water or oil. A number of diseases are treated by applying electromagnets. Magnetic water is also used for balancing the polarisation of the body.

21. Chromotherapy

The seven colsrs of the sun are utilized through radiation on the body or by directing charged oil or water for treatment.

22. Reiki

This form of naturopathy is used to balance chakras and energy

23. Water Therapy

Water is the most ancient of all the remedial agents. It is employed in different forms in treatment and produces several types of physiological effects depending upon temperature and duration. Hydrotherapy is employed in almost all types of disease conditions.

24. Air Therapy

Fresh air is essential for good health. Air therapy is employed in different pressures and temp. in variety of disease conditions.

25. Fire Therapy

Existence of all the creatures and forms depends upon "Agni" (Fire). In Nature Cure treatment, different temperatures are employed through different heating techniques to produce different specific effects.

26. Space Therapy

Congestion causes disease. Fasting is the best therapy to relieve congestion of body and mind

27. Chromotherapy

Sun rays have seven colours – violet, indigo, blue, green, yellow, orange and red. These colours are employed through irradiation or body or by administering charged water, oil and pills for treatment.

28. Naturopathic Obstetrics

Naturopathic physicians provide natural childbirth care in an out-of-hospital setting. They offer prenatal and postnatal care using modern diagnostic techniques. The naturopathic approach strengthens healthy body functions so that complications associated with pregnancy may be prevented.

29. Oriental Medicine

Oriental medicine is a complimentary healing philosophy to naturopathic medicine. The meridian theory offers an important understanding of the unity of the body and mind, and adds to the Western understanding of physiology. Acupuncture provides a method of treatment which can unify and harmonise the imbalances present in disease conditions, which, if untreated, can result in illness.

30. Psychological Medicine

Mental attitudes and emotional states may influence, or even cause, physical illness. Counseling, nutritional balancing, stress management, hypnotherapy, biofeedback and other therapies are used to help patients heal on the psychological level.

Naturopaths consider patients to be participants in their health care, so you may be asked to make lifestyle changes (such as chaning your sleeping, eating, and exercise habits).

Naturopathic philosophy serves as the basis for naturopathic practice. The current scope of naturopathic practice includes, but is not limited to, the following:

Clinical Nutrition

A cornerstone of naturopathic practice is that food is the best medicine. The relationship between nutrition and wellness, or between inadequate nutrition and disease, is well documented and is a cornerstone of naturopathic practice.

Naturopathic application of clinical nutrition involves the use of dietetics and specific nutritional substances for the prevention and treatment of disease, the correction of dietary inadequacies and the promotion of wellness. Many medical conditions can be treated more effectively with foods and nutritional supplements than by other means, with fewer complications and side effects.

Many pharmaceuticals can be strengthened and targeted more safely with knowledge of nutritional sciences. Naturopathic physicians use dietetics, natural hygiene, fasting and nutritional supplementation in their practice. These methods can be used as either alternatives to mainstream medicine, or as complementary and in concert with it, depending on the desires of the patient.

Botanical Medicine

Plant. substances have been utilised safely and effectively for centuries in the prevention and treatment of diseases. Their clinical uses and effects are described in detail in traditional literature, and they are the subject of an increasing amount of new scientific research.

Many plant substances are powerful medicines. Whereas a single chemically derived drug may address a single problem, botanical medicines are able to address a variety of problems simultaneously.

Documentation exists that demonstrates the safe and effective use of many botanical medicines over generations. Their organic nature makes botanicals compatible with the body's own chemistry; hence, they can be gently effective with fewer toxic side effects.

Their availability and safety make them more useful and affordable for home care of chronic conditions. Botanical medicines have pharmacological properties that necessitate their use by appropriately trained health care providers.

Naturopathic Obstetrics

Naturopathic physicians provide natural childbirth care in either an out-of-hospital setting, or in a hospital. They offer prenatal and postnatal care using modern diagnostic techniques.

The naturopathic approach strengthens healthy body functions so that complications associated with pregnancy can be prevented or minimised.

Homoeopathic Medicine

Homoeopathic medicine was originally developed during the 18th century by the German physician Hahnemann, and is widely used throughout the world. Minute amounts of substances prepared and prescribed according to strict homoeopathic principles are used to evoke a physiological and/or psychological response.

Homoeopathic medicine is based on the principle of "like cures like". It works on a subtle yet powerful electromagnetic level, gently acting to strengthen the body's healing and immune response. Because these are both effective and very safe, naturopathic physicians share a respect for this system of medicine with practitioners of many other healing arts.

Homoeopathy is a central part of our comprehensive training for these reasons. The practice of homoeopathic medicine includes a unique and detailed method of case taking and analysis, and an indepth knowledge of homoeopathic *materia medicals.*

Physical Medicine

Naturopathic medicine has traditionally utilised a wide variety of physical modalities for the treatment of pain and to stimulate circulation and healing.

Naturopathic medicine has its own methods of therapeutic manipulation of muscles, bones, and the spine. These include heat/cold, light, ultraviolet and infrared, electrical pulsation, magnetic field, therapeutic ultrasound, diathermy, interferential, cold laser, hydrotherapy, colon therapy, traction, massage and exercise. The physicians also use ultrasound, diathermy, exercise, massage, water, heat and cold, air, and gentle electrical pulses to treat acute or chronic physical injury.

Many recent advances in sports medicine and exercise physiology are essentially adaptations of herbal and homoeopathic materials into the modern arena.

Oriental Medicine

Oriental medicine and acupuncture comprise a unique system that has been in use for 5,000 years for the diagnosis and treatment of disease. This system employs unique methods for evaluating the flow and balance of energy in the body, and includes the specialised use of Oriental herbs and acupuncture. Naturopathic doctors are trained to use this system when indicated as part of an integrated approach with Western diagnostic methods.

Oriental medicine is a complementary philosophy of natural healing brought to the medical community, largely through naturopathic medicine. Asiatic and Oriental systems offer an important understanding of the unity of the body and mind, which add to those of the West. Unification between philosophy and practice in the East and West offers health benefits for all of our cultures.

Chinese medicine and ayurveda provide ancient understandings and methods of treatment. These promise to help harmonise the imbalances present in disease conditions and restore the dynamic balance of health.

Psychological Medicine

A tenet of naturopathic medicine is that emotional health and physical health are interdependent. Naturopathic practice includes the integrated use of counseling techniques along with such methods as stress management and biofeedback when indicated. Mental attitudes and emotional states may influence, or even cause, physical illness.

Counselling, nutritional balancing, stress management, hypnotherapy, biofeedback, and other therapies are used to help patients heal on levels other than only the physical.

Minor Surgery

As general practitioners, naturopathic physicians do in-office minor surgery, including repair of superficial wounds, removal of foreign bodies, cysts, and other superficial masses. We refer to surgeons when their skills are needed for our patient's well-being.

Lifestyle Modification and Public Health

Environment and lifestyle have a significant impact on health. Contamination of food, water or the local environment, and extremes in diet can cause a significant risk for the patient. These factors are evaluated and dealt with when appropriate.

Mechanotherapy including Manipulation of the Spine and Extremities

Mechanotherapy includes both the manipulation and mobilisation of the joints of the spine and extremities, as well as other physical and mechanical techniques applied to connective tissue.

Mechanotherapy has been part of naturopathic medicine since the turn of the century and is used in conjunction with one or more other naturopathic modalities.

These are the major areas that most naturopathic physicians' practices include.

The naturopathic philosophy and approach to disease are all-encompassing, and naturopaths treat most illnesses. Naturopaths can and do diagnose, apply naturopathic therapy to, and thereby treat, acute infectious disease and abnormalities of the digestive system, the respiratory system, the cardiovascular system, the urinary system, the hemopoetic system, the nervous system and the endocrine system.

Although naturopathic physicians treat patients of all ages, they treat a high proportion of geriatric patients.

The diagnostic aids used by naturopaths include every accepted diagnostic instrument: sphygmomanometer; stethoscope; electrocardiograph; endocardiograph; thermometer; speculums; proctoscope; sigmoidoscopes; instruments for testing, reflexes, aural receptivity, and for testing pressure of eyeball; scales, X-ray; fluoroscopes — the gamut of modern medicine's diagnostic equipment.

Some naturopaths undertake "iridiagnosis" as part of their diagnostic evaluations. It is based on the belief that bodily departures from the normal cause observable markings in the eyes of the patient. By study of these markings, according to basic naturopathy, the naturopath can learn a complete history of past illnesses, as well as previous treatment. For example, drugs taken by the patient are said to cause appearance of certain markings and colours at a later time. Such unnatural treatment always leaves more signs and markings in the iris than were there before the treatment. Under naturopathic treatment the disease signs lessen or completely disappear.

Naturopathy does, in general, rely less heavily on radical alteration of bodily functions and chemistry than do other healing arts. Its primary stresses include light therapy; electrotherapy; vibrotherapy; remedial exercises; manipulations; vasomotor control; mechanical therapy; chemotherapy; biochemic therapy, phytotherapy — using naturopathic botanicals, herbal, and vegetable materials; the use of tissue minerals and cell salts; vapotherapy; colon therapy — irrigating agents and other products for the treatment pathoses of this region; autotherapies; climatotherapy.

Treatment Methods

Emphasis is placed upon nutritional advice and elimination of waste. The following treatment methods are cited as examples:

Treatment of Retention

Opening the pores of the skin, increasing respiration, increasing excretion of the kidneys, supplying adequate ingestion of proper minerals, particularly. Food is withheld during the acute stages.

Treatment of Invasion

Opening the pores of the skin, general tonic treatment to control and only to keep the symptoms within safe limits. Congenial germicides may be used.

Treatment for Enervation

General tonic treatments to maintain adequate circulation, adequate nutrition. Usually this will require some of the mineral phosphates and quite often vitamins in large doses. Also securing emotional rest and stimulating the skin and other emunctories

The naturopath attempts to prevent morbid matter or toxins from accumulating by prescribing pure, natural foods. Eating flesh and drinking coffee or tea, the "multiple barrelled poison", are discouraged. Naturopaths believe that the extensive use of flesh meats may lead to auto-intoxication, a resultant of decomposition or decay of undigested remnants, and cause intestinal catarrh, ulceration, biliousness, appendicitis, and many other diseases

It is apparent that naturopaths' approach to health and disease is very different from that of medicine and osteopathy.

What Practitioners do in Treating Patients

A first visit to a naturopathic practitioner is usually an extended appointment. The practitioner will interview the patient at length about his health history, reasons for the visit, and lifestyle (such as diet, stress, alcohol and tobacco use, sleep, and exercise). The practitioner may perform examinations and, if in her scope of practice, order diagnostic and screening tests. Toward the end of the appointment, a management plan is set up to address the patient's general health and problems with illness. Referrals to other health care providers may be made, if appropriate. Practitioners may deliver some naturopathic treatments in their offices, such as hydrotherapy or manipulation.

Examples of additional treatments are:

1. Dietary changes (for example, eating more whole and unprocessed foods)
2. Vitamins, minerals, and other dietary supplements
3. Herbal medicine
4. Counselling and education on lifestyle changes
5. Homoeopathy
6. Hydrotherapy (for example, applying hot water, then cold water)
7. Manual and body-based therapies such as manipulation and mobilisation
8. Exercise therapy
9. Mind-body therapies such as yoga and meditation.
10. A conscious mental process using certain techniques, such as focusing attention or maintaining a specific posture, to suspend the stream of thoughts and relax the body and mind.

Some practitioners use other treatments as well.

Natural Treatment

There are several naturally found materials in India that offer economical natural treatments through naturopathy. Some of these are the lemon, milk and salt.

Lemon and Naturopathy

For cough, cold and fever, lemon is very effective. Squeeze a lemon in a glass full of water and drink repeatedly. This will cure all of the three ailments. But if the fever is high and makes one thirsty, boil the water. This will bring down the fever and reduce the thirst. If the cold is severe, it can be added to the required amount of honey in the above mixture. Another very beneficial method is as follows: cut a lemon in half, add in it salt, ground black pepper and powdered molasses.

Heat this and squeeze the juice directly on the tongue. To remove the freckles on the face, rub a piece of lemon on them and they will lighten considerably. Sprinkling a little alum on the lemon works wonders for the complexion. Rubbing half a lemon on the teeth not only makes the teeth shiny and bright but will also cure bad breath. To reduce the body weight adds a little salt and one lemon to 350 ml of lukewarm water and drink daily on an empty stomach. You can also substitute honey to salt.

Milk and Naturopathy

Milk should ideally be consumed in the morning since it is believed that the heat of the sun helps in digestion of milk. Adding sugar to milk is very harmful since it not only induces phlegm, it also destroys the calcium content in it. It should be drunk at room temperature if possible. However, if one prefers warm milk, then do not overheat it.

Overheating destroys all its beneficial elements. For the sweetening of milk and easy digestion, one can add honey to it. If one is suffering from cough, constipation, diarrhola, stomachache, or indigestion, he/she should avoid consumption of milk. For acidity, drink cold milk twice a day. For hiccups, it is advised to warm a glass of milk and drink. In addition, for tiredness, a glass of warm milk will prove effective. For wrinkles, pimples and blemishes, warm milk can be applied.

After half an hour, wash the face with clean water. One has to do it regularly before sleeping at night; then it will solve the problem and improve the complexion. Adding a little saffron to a spoonful of fresh milk and applying it on the lips will cure their darkness and make them softer. If one is suffering from an itchy rash, add a little water to some milk and apply on the rash with cotton wool and then wash. It will stop the itch and cure the rash.

Salt and Naturopathy

Salt is good only in small quantities and rock salt is better than sea salt. Eating excessive salt weakens the gums and is also the cause of body odour. Due to excessive consumption of salt, body cells die, and when these dead cells come out through the pores with perspiration, the odor is very strong and foul. To help the situation, one can consume salt in very small quantities. Salt is very drying; hence, excessive amounts of salt will cause unnatural thirst. But it can be very beneficial as well.

In a headache, keep a pinch of salt on the tongue or smell a mixture of three grams of salt in one-fourth cup of water. For a stomachache, mix half a spoon salt in a glass of hot water and drink. This will not only cure the pain but will also remove the cause of the pain. For softening the skin, wet the skin and take a fistful of salt and rub in circular motions and then wash. It is advised to do it once a week and it will slough off dead skin, thus making it soft. For cracking heels or rough feet, soak the feet in warm water by adding some salt to it.

Various Fields of Naturopathy

The focus of naturopathy is on its philosophy of natural self-healing rather than specific methods, and practitioners use a wide variety of treatment modalities. The particular modalities utilised by an individual naturopath varies with training and scope of practice. The demonstrated efficacy and scientific rationale also vary. These include:

1. Acupressure
2. Acupuncture
3. Applied Kinesiology
4. Aromatherapy
5. Bach Flower Therapy
6. Chiropractic
7. Chromotherapy
8. Homoeopathy

9. Magneto Therapy
10. Massage Therapy
11. Mud Therapy
12. Ozone Therapy
13. Reflexology
14. Traditional Chinese Medicine
15. Rolfing
16. Water Therapy

There are other nature cure therapies, such as, botanical medicine, chelation therapy for atherosclerosis, colonic enemas, cranial osteopathy, hair analysis, iridology, physical medicine, psychological counselling (examples include meditation, relaxation and other methods of stress management), etc., but we shall deal with only the above-stated ones.

5

Acupressure

Acupressure is an ancient healing art that uses the fingers to press key points on the surface of the skin to stimulate the body's natural self-curative abilities. When these points are pressed, they release muscular tension and promote the circulation of blood and the body's life force to aid healing.

Various techniques applied in an acupressure treatment include pressing, rubbing, gentle stretching, and rolling, chafing, kneading, wiping and grasping, as well as corrective exercises. Varying levels of pressure are used, most often starting by applying light pressure and gradually working deeper. The practitioner may focus more energy or pressure on a specific point or series of points, depending on the individual's chief complaint, or the entire course of a meridian may be addressed.

Various techniques applied in an acupressure treatment include pressing, rubbing, gentle stretching, and rolling, chafing, kneading, wiping and grasping, as well as corrective exercises. Varying levels of pressure are used, most often starting by applying light pressure and gradually working deeper. The practitioner may focus more energy or pressure on a specific point or series of points, depending on the individual's chief complaint, or the entire course of a meridian may be addressed.

Acupuncture and Acupressure

Acupuncture and acupressure use the same points, but acupuncture employs needles, while acupressure uses the gentle but firm pressure of hands (and even feet). There is a massive amount of scientific data that demonstrates why and how acupuncture is effective. But acupressure, the older of the two traditions, was neglected after the Chinese developed more technological methods for stimulating points with needles and electricity. Acupressure, however, continues to be the most effective method for self-treatment of tension-related ailments by using the power and sensitivity of the human hand.

Acupuncture is based on the theory that there is an invisible force or energy in nature that the Chinese call qi. According to the principles of traditional Chinese medicine, the body has vital energy called *chi* or *qi* that flows along invisible lines of energy flow called meridians. In a manner similar to blood circulation, *qi* flows to each cell via a complex network of pathways usually called 'channels' or'meridians'.

If *qi* gets stuck, it causes an imbalance as upstream cells are flooded with too much *qi* and downstream cells receive too little. Acupuncture points are those spots where *qi* has the greatest tendency to get stuck; hence stimulating them with needles (acupuncture) or finger pressure (acupressure) helps free stuck *qi* and restore normal circulation. Once normal qi circulation is restored, the cells eventually return to their normal, healthy state.

There are thought to be at least 14 meridians connecting our organs with other parts of our body. Acupuncture and acupressure points lie on those meridians. If the flow of *qi* is blocked at any point on a meridian, it's thought to be the cause of ailments and lead to disease anywhere along the meridian. That's why a practitioner may apply pressure to an acupressure point in the foot to relieve a headache.

Acupressure therapy is performed on the same acupuncture points that are used to stimulate the flow of *qi* and *xue*. After repeated acupressure sessions using different degrees of pressure, you will begin to feel a pulse at the point. This pulsation is a good sign - it means that circulation has increased. Pay attention to the type of pulse you feel. If it's very faint or throbbing, hold the point longer until the pulse balances.

The body and all matter is made up of electro-magnetic forces. It was ironically Western scientists who ingeniously verified the existence of electromagnetism which provided a logical explanation for the positive results from acupuncture and acupressure therapy. It has a rapport with the energy of the body and can travel through the body like other forms of electricity, sound, and waveforms of energy. When needles or pressure are used, they act as antennae that conduct the electromagnetic energy from the air into the body. Acupressure massage can be very effective both as prevention and as a treatment for many health conditions. Acupressure techniques have been used to provide quick, cost-free, and effective relief from many symptoms.

Benefits of Acupressure

1. Foremost among the advantages of acupressure's healing touch is that it is safe to do on yourself and others - even if you've never done it before - so long as you follow the instructions and pay attention to the cautions.
2. There are no side effects from drugs, because there are no drugs. And the only equipment needed is your own two hands.
3. You can practise acupressure therapy any time, anywhere.
4. *Acupressure* can be effective in helping relieve headaches, eyestrain, sinus problems, neck pain, backaches, arthritis, muscle aches and tension due to stress.

5. *Acupressure* also helps to relieve ulcer pain, menstrual cramps, lower back aches, constipation and indigestion.
6. You can also use self-acupressure to relieve anxiety and to help you get to sleep at night.
7. In acupressure, local symptoms are considered an expression of the condition of the body as a whole.
8. A tension headache, for instance, may be rooted in the shoulder and neck area. Thus acupressure focuses on relieving pain and discomfort as well as on responding to tension before it develops into a "disease", that is, before the constrictions and imbalances can do further damage.
9. By using a combination of self-help methods such as trigger point stimulation, deep breathing, range-of-motion exercises, and relaxation techniques, you can improve your condition as well as feel more alive, healthy, and in harmony with your life.

There is no scientific consensus on how acupressure might work. Some theorise that the pressure may promote the release of natural pain-relieving chemicals in the body, called endorphins. Another theory is that the pressure may somehow influence the autonomic nervous system.

Common Ailments Curable by Acupressure

Most people try acupressure for a specific ailment. Some of the more common ailments are:

1. Nausea and vomiting during pregnancy/ morning sickness
2. Motion sickness
3. Nausea after surgery
4. Nausea due to chemotherapy
5. Cancer-related fatigue
6. Headache

7. Menstrual cramps
8. Muscle tension and pain

Although more research is needed, studies examining the use of acupressure for nausea have generally found that it's effective at relieving nausea.

Application of Acupressure

Acupressure is often administered by an acupuncturist with the person receiving the acupressure lying on a massage table. Acupressure can also be self-administered. Although it's best to consult an acupuncturist for proper instruction, acupressure is generally done by using the thumb, finger or knuckle to apply gentle but firm pressure to a point. The pressure is often increased for about 30 seconds, held steadily for 30 seconds to two minutes and then gradually decreased for 30 seconds. It's often repeated three to five times.

The Don'ts of Acupressure

1. Acupressure should never be painful. If you experience any pain, discontinue the session.
2. Pressure should be gentle over fragile or sensitive areas, such as the face.
3. People with osteoporosis, recent fracture or injury, easy bruising, bleeding disorders, circulatory problems from diabetes, and those using anticoagulant or antiplatelet that "thin" the blood should avoid acupressure unless under the supervision of a qualified therapist.
4. Pregnant women should consult their doctor before using acupressure. Acupressure shouldn't be done on the abdominal area or to certain points on the leg if pregnant.
5. Acupressure shouldn't be done over open wounds, bruises, varicose veins, or any area that is bruised or swollen.
6. After an acupressure session, some people may feel soreness at the points. People may also feel temporarily lightheaded.

There are also great advantages to using acupressure as a way to balance the body and maintain good health. The healing touch of acupressure reduces tension, increases circulation, and enables the body to relax deeply. By relieving stress, acupressure strengthens resistance to disease and promotes wellness

There are, however, a number of points that are useful for acupressure in the sense that they are easy to apply acupressure techniques with and they have generally useful and precise functions that do not require a more developed diagnosis before use.

Hand Chart

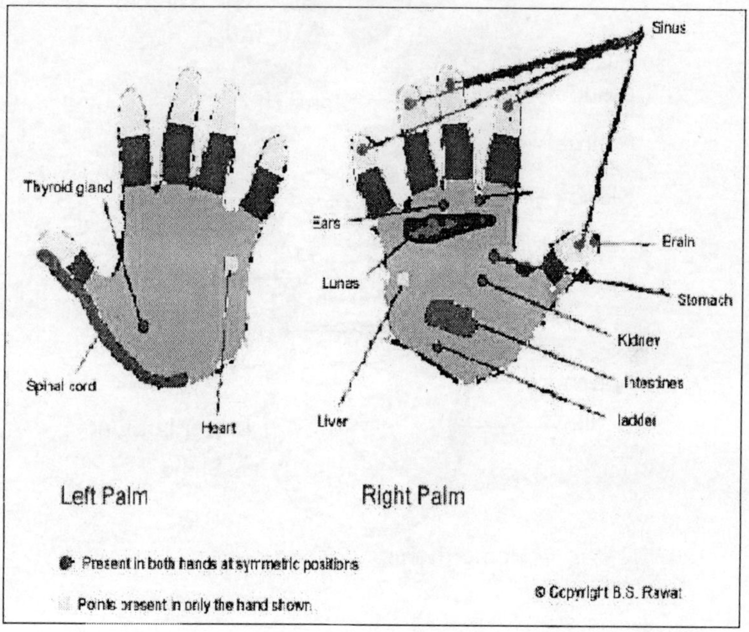

Foot chart

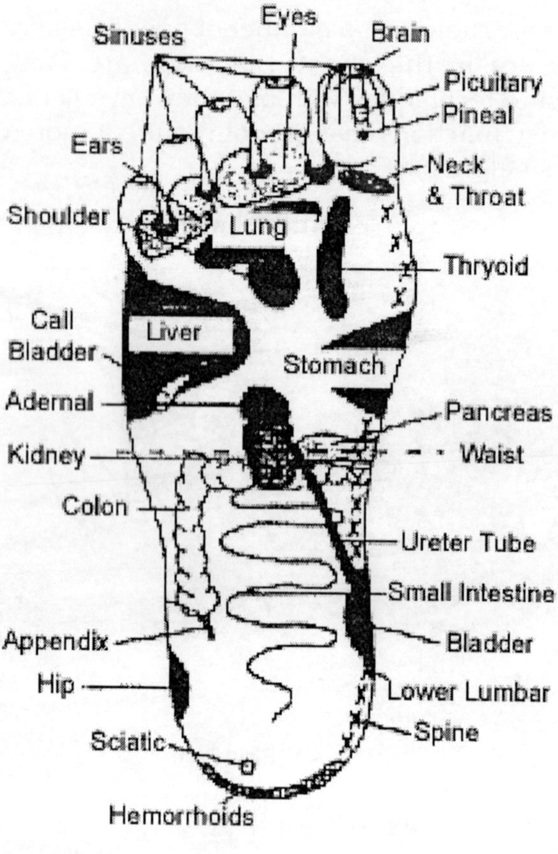

Eyes
Sinuses
Brain
Picuitary
Pineal
Ears
Neck
& Throat
Shoulder
Lung
Thryoid
Call
Bladder
Liver
Stomach
Adernal
Pancreas
Kidney
Waist
Colon
Ureter Tube
Small Intestine
Appendix
Bladder
Hip
Lower Lumbar
Spine
Sciatic
Hemorrhoids

6
Acupuncture

What is Acupuncture?

Acupuncture is an element of Traditional Chinese Medicine (TCM) that originated in China more than 2,000 years ago. It is one of the oldest and most commonly used medical procedures in the world. Based on natural law and energy, acupuncture is a complex system of diagnostic corollaries that treat the person as a whole rather than only focusing on specific isolated symptoms.

The word acupuncture comes from the Latin acus, "needle", and pungere, "to prick".

Acupuncture therapy is a holistic form of health care, rooted in the ancient philosophy known as Daoism, which concentrates on the need for change, growth, balance and harmony. In recent years there has been increased scientific research into the benefits of acupuncture-based therapies, and this forms a fundamental part of the current trend towards complementary therapy in Western society.

Most of the acupuncturists suggest the traditional Chinese view of health and disease. An acupuncture therapy along with herbal remedies and other related ways are considered as valid approaches in curing your disease.

Yin and Yang

The essence of acupuncture is to balance *yin* and *yang* inorder to keep the normal flow of energy unblocked. Acupuncture is also used to maintain or restore health to the body and mind by stimulating the body's natural healing abilities. Because of its ability to promote healing in the body it has been proven beneficial to those in eating disorder treatment centres and for those seeking treatment for drug abuse.

Role of Needles in Acupuncture

Acupuncture therapy involves insertion of very thin, stainless steel needles into various parts of your body. To produce better stimulation, low frequency electric currents are also applied to the needles. Acupuncture treatment involves stimulation of points on the body by penetrating the skin with metallic, hair-thin needles. Needles placed into the body vary in amount and depth reached. Each needle can stay in place for as long as an hour, but the typical time length is approximately 25 minutes.

Twirling, warming and electronic energising are not uncommon in acupuncture, and can intensify the session. If electricity is the effect chosen, a light prickling sensation will follow, increasing or decreasing in strength depending on the acupuncturist and your own preferences.

Acupuncture therapy is an effective means of stimulating acupoints with lasers, ultrasound and electricity.

Other Procedures Used with Acupuncture

The procedures which can also be used in conjunction with acupuncture therapy are:

1. Auriculotherapy - Placement of needles in the ear
2. *Acupressure* - Use of manual pressure
3. Moxibustion - Burning of floss or herbs which are applied to the skin
4. Procaine
5. Injection of sterilised water
6. Vitamins
7. Morphine

8. Homoeopathic solutions which are inserting through the needles

Acupuncture Points

Acupuncture therapy is applied to the acupuncture points which are supposed to be located throughout your body. During the past 2,000 years there were 365 points located which represented as the days of the year. Gradually this number has increased to around 2,000.

The vital energy or *chi/qi* in your body flows through channels, which are known as meridians. TCM theorises that there are nearly 2,000 acupuncture points on the human body which are connected by 12 main meridians and eight extraordinary pathways.

Meridians consist of branches which connect to bodily organs or functions. Any imbalance to these *chi* levels is considered as illness. These meridians which run just beneath the skin conduct energy or *Qi* throughout the body. *Qi*, the life force, regulates spiritual, emotional, mental and physical balance, and is influenced by *yin* and *yang*, a concept of opposing qualities which can cause illness when they become imbalanced. The ancient practices such as acupuncture therapy, herbal therapy and *qi gong* exercise are the main considerations to restore the imbalance in your body.

Factors Responsible for Imbalance of Equili-brium

There are many factors that can upset the natural balance of *Qi*, including emotional states such as anxiety, stress, anger, fear or grief, and particularly when they are suppressed, as they so often are in modern society.

Many other factors including nutrition, physical environment, hereditary constitution, infections or other physical trauma including surgery, can all contribute towards the imbalance of natural equilibrium. Acupuncture therapy aims, by the use of fine needles inserted into carefully selected points along these meridians, to re-establish the body's energetic harmony.

Twelve Main Meridians

The 12 meridians are separated into *yin* and *yang*, with various meridians on the legs and arms. Each meridian represents a biological function in the body and thus may not be anatomically placed.

1. Lung
2. Large intestine
3. Stomach
4. Spleen
5. Heart
6. Small intestine
7. Urinary bladder
8. Kidney
9. Pericardium
10. Triple warmer
11. Gall bladder
12. Liver

Benefits of Acupuncture

Can acupuncture benefit healthy people? Many people use acupuncture in order to prevent illness. It is also used as a way of keeping the immune system healthy.

1. Acupuncture pain management brings both physical and emotional relief to those suffering from both acute and chronic discomfort as it is best know for controlling pain.
2. It has also been helpful for those in drug rehab facilities, bulimia centres, anorexia treatment facilities and for those seeking help with various psychological disorders.
3. Mental clarity is another benefit of acupuncture. This is because acupuncture helps to balance the body's natural flow of energy.
4. Acupuncture therapy can cure chronic pain in the neck and back.

5. Acupuncture therapy can cure behavioral problems.
6. Acupuncture therapy can cure migraines and headaches.
7. It can cure ligament and muscle tear.
8. It can cure genito-urinary conditions.
9. It can cure problems with the stomach and intestine.
10. It can cure muscle and nerve problems.
11. It can cure injury related pain such as strains.
12. It can cure cardiovascular conditions.

Diagnosis before Conducting Acupuncture Therapy

The diagnosis of a patient includes many things like:

a. Patient's medical history and lifestyle
b. Examining the skin and tongue
c. Listening to breathing sounds
d. Pulse recording

The electrical properties in your body can become imbalanced several weeks or months before the physical symptoms occur.

Side Effects of Acupuncture Therapy

a. Harm to internal organs.
b. Improper sterilisation of the needles can cause infection.
c. Weakening of your body's system due to the reaction of needles.
d. Bleeding in the needle inserted areas.

The World Health Organisation has recognised and defined acupuncture points and procedures as a safe and effective alternative therapy.

Acupuncture points are mapped to fourteen major meridians.

One meridian is present at one of the twelve internal organs and in remaining two, one is present along spine and another is present along midline of abdomen.

Recently many extra points are determined in different parts of body such as nose, ears, scalp, hands wrist, feet and ankles.

The different acupuncture points present in different meridians are as follows:

1. *Acupuncture point present in large intestine meridian:* The point present in large intestine meridian point is present between thumb and first finger on the back side of hand. This acupuncture point is used in the treatment of feverish diseases and inflammatory diseases and if you have symptoms in throat and head. The large intestine meridian passes through head and hand. This acupuncture point is used for determining upper body disorders. The upper body disorders include sore throat, eye pain, rashes and difficulty in moving arms. This acupuncture point also determines intestinal disorders such as diarrhea and intestinal cramping.
2. *Acupuncture point present in lung meridian:* The point present in lung meridian is present inside the arm that is above wrist. This point is used for determining upper body disorders such as head ache, neck stiffness, asthma, cough, sore throat, facial paralysis and problems in wrist.
3. *Acupuncture point present in stomach meridian:* The point present in stomach meridian is located in front of leg that is just below knee. This point is used for determining stomach disorders such as nausea, vomiting and abdominal distension. This is also used for determining general weakness. Acupuncture point present in stomach meridian also demonstrates positive effects in treating anemia, immune deficiency, fatigue and many other diseases.
4. *Acupuncture point in spleen meridian:* This point is present just above the ankle at the inner side of the leg. These points are used for treating hormonal disorders and immune disorders.

5. *Acupuncture point present in gall bladder meridian:* This point is present at the base of skull where it joins the neck back side. This point is used in treating mild disorders such as cold, influenza, neck pain and fever. It is also used for lowering blood pressures and relaxes tension.

Acupuncture is a therapy which promotes health and elevates pain and suffering and it helps to heal within coherent system and also known as oriental medicine. Sometimes you might be confused with the symptoms that with which disease you are affected. At this time, acupuncture points help you.

❖❖❖

7

Applied Kinesiology

What is Kinesiology?

Kinesiology is the study of the various disciplines that encompass the movement of the human body.

Kinesiology, literally the study of body movement, originated in the 1960's, and combines Western techniques with Eastern wisdom to promote physical, emotional and spiritual health.

Kinesiology is defined primarily as the use of muscle testing to identify imbalances in the body's structural, chemical, emotional or other energy, to establish the body's priority healing needs, and to evaluate energy changes brought about by a broad spectrum of both manual and non-manual therapeutic procedures.

Put simply, kinesiology is a non-invasive method using muscle feedback and body awareness, that can help you to reduce stress and pain, improve performance at school, work and home, in sports, in relationships, and promote health and well-being.

Kinesiology may either be pure or applied. Pure kinesiology seeks to understand human movement in order to analyse problems and come up with treatments for these problems. Applied kinesiology is a specific method to treat these problems.

Kinesiology is defined primarily as the use of muscle testing to identify imbalances in the body's structural, chemical, emotional or other energy, to establish the body's priority healing needs, and to evaluate energy changes brought about by a broad spectrum of both manual and non-manual therapeutic procedures.

Kinesiology, therefore, may be understood as a system of natural health care which combines muscle monitoring with the principles of Chinese medicine to assess energy and body function, applying a range of gentle yet powerful healing techniques to improve health, well being and vitality.

Kinesiology is not a single discipline. Rather, it is an umbrella class of study which covers many different disciplines. The primary focuses of kinesiology are human physiology, biomechanics and anatomy. A study of kinesiology may also cover the psychology, philosophy, ecology and even sociology of sports and exercise.

How Does It Work?

Kinesiologists have found that many things (including mental stress or fears, our diet and daily exercise) affect muscle balance, and hence our energy levels, posture and the way we function and feel. When all aspects of our lives are balanced, the best results follow and we function at our vital best. Kinesiology uses feedback from muscle testing to identify and eliminate different forms of stress.

Precision muscle monitoring techniques are applied to identify and correct energy blockages within the body.

Always the answer is somewhere inside you. Muscle monitoring is a natural feedback system using an indicator muscle, which supplies information via nerve pathways and the meridian system of the brain and body.

Kinesiology bypasses conscious thinking processes to isolate causal factors in the subconscious, body and etheric levels. Honouring this system enables the body to clear itself at its own enhanced rate and priority.

A fundamental premise of kinesiology is that the body has innate healing energy and is at all times doing its best to care for itself, but that sometimes it needs to be helped into a better position to achieve this care.

Kinesiology also recognises that there are flows of energy within the body that relate not only to the muscles but to every tissue and organ that go to make the body a living, feeling being.

These energy flows can be evaluated by testing the function of the muscles, which in turn reflect the body's overall state of structural, chemical or emotional balance. In this way, kinesiology taps into energies that the more conventional modalities overlook.

Kinesiology looks beyond the symptoms. It does not treat named diseases. Nor does it diagnose them. It is concerned with imbalances in the body's energy. In this respect, kinesiology has close links with the acupuncture concept of energy flow.

Kinesiology is not limited to dealing with ailments. Energy balancing brings a person closer to achieving any goal of their choice — in sport, relationships, learning or coping with life in general.

Kinesiology is a non-invasive method, using precision muscle feedback and body awareness that can help you to reduce stress and pain, improve performance at school, work and home, in sports, in relationships, and promotes health and well being. It helps one access the inner knowing and discover again the power of choice in one's life.

Kinesiology identifies factors which block the body's natural healing processes. These dysfunctions are rectified by attention to reflex and acupressure points, the use of specific body movements and nutritional support.

In general, the applied kinesiologist finds a muscle that tests as weak, and then attempts to determine why that muscle is not functioning properly. The practitioner will then evaluate and apply the therapy that will best eliminate the muscle weakness and help the patient.

Benefits of Kinesiology

1. Kinesiology can relieve pain, stress, muscular and nervous disorders, detect allergies and nutritional deficiencies, assist with psychological and learning problems, stimulate energies and release untapped potential.
2. One of the great advantages in using applied kinesiology is the ability to affect performance. Examples of this range from increasing the breathing capacity in endurance athletes, to increasing the accuracy of those sports requiring eye-hand or eye-foot coordination.

Therapies Used

Therapies utilised can include specific joint manipulation or mobilisation, various myofacial therapies, cranial techniques, meridian therapy, clinical nutrition, dietary management and various reflex procedures.

In some cases, the examiner may test for environmental or food sensitivities by using a previously strong muscle to find what weakens it.

Applied Kinesiology

Applied kinesiology uses the triad of health - chemical, mental and structural factors - to describe the proper balance of the major health categories. The triad is represented by an equilateral triangle with structural health as its base, and the upright sides representing chemical and mental health. When a person experiences poor health, it is due to an imbalance in one or more of these three factors.

The triad of health is interactive and all sides must be evaluated for the underlying cause of a problem. A health problem on one side of the triad can affect the other sides. For example, a chemical imbalance may cause mental symptoms. Applied kinesiology enables the practitioner to evaluate the triad's balance and direct the therapy toward the imbalanced side or sides.

George Goodheart,the founder of applied kinesiology, was the first chiropractor named to the United States Olympic Medical Team in 1980. Since then, many other doctors in countries around the world have helped athletes in the Olympics. Doctors using applied kinesiology have been and continue to be important assets to professional baseball, basketball, football, hockey and soccer teams.

Healing of strain-sprain type injuries goes through three distinct processes. Each requires special tools to maximise the return to normal functioning.

The first is termed the reaction phase and usually lasts up to seven days. This is where there is the most pain and swelling. Treatment must reduce the swelling and pain and prevent further damage while the body begins to clean up and remove damaged tissue. Important issues here are diet, activation of lymphatic drainage and control of inflammatory processes.

The second stage is called the regeneration phase and can start as early as two days after the injury and take upto eight plus weeks. In this stage, the body rebuilds the damaged tissues. This is done through creation of a matrix of collagen. During this stage, treatment is aimed at making strong bonds and increasing normal actions in the joints. Special procedures can be used here to speed the rebuilding, start to reestablish lost strength and increase the range of motion and control of muscle function.

The final stage of healing is the remodeling phase. During this phase, muscles must fully regain their lost strength. Other important aspects are the coordination of muscular actions as well as reestablishing a full range of motion. Depending on the severity of injury, this phase starts as early as the 14th day and can take over a year. During this phase, therapies are used that are aimed at normalizing proprioception imbalances in the muscles and joint structures. A special use of muscle testing, used at this time, is to determine exactly how much you should exercise a muscle so that you are reinjuring yourself.

Through the skills learned in courses on applied kinesiology, these doctors are able to tailor a treatment programme to speed recovery and maximise performance.

❖❖❖

8

Aromatherapy

What is Aromatherapy?

Aromatherapy is the practice of using volatile plant oils, including essential oils, for psychological and physical well being. It is the ancient science of healing, relaxing and energising by the use of plants and their parts. The roots, barks, flowers, fruits, seeds and nuts play a crucial part in this science. It is one of the more popular branches of alternative medicines.

The word 'aromatherapy' is derived from two words: *aroma* which means smell, and *therapy* which stands for healing. The history of aromatherapy essential oils dates back to centuries ago to ancient civilisations such as those of Egypt, India, China and Greece.

Different cultures had different uses for essential fragrant oils, and while aromatherapy candles had not yet been developed, ancient aromatherapy products in India included herb-based incense sticks that were used for religious practices.

Aromatherapies are often used for their medicinal effects. But aroma therapists might soon have a new career as alternative psychiatrists.

Essential Oils

Essential oils form the basis of aromatherapy. These essentials oils are the extracts of plants and their parts, and form their life force. These oils are extracted by the means of steam distillation, cold expression, or fixed oil or alcohol extraction. The distiller is necessary because plants degrade when cooked at high temperatures. Essential oil distillers were invented by a chemist named Ibn Sina for the creation of drinks and perfumes.

Products that include synthetic ingredients are frowned upon in holistic aromatherapy. It is important to note that perfume oils also known as fragrance oils (and usually listed as "fragrance" on an ingredient label) are not the same as essential oils. Fragrance oils and perfume oils contain synthetic chemicals and do not provide the therapeutic benefits of essential oils.

There are quite a few products on the market that contain unnatural ingredients including fragrance oils and claim to be aromatherapeutic. It's important to look at the ingredient label when seeking true aromatherapy products. Also, use caution with marketing claims that state a product is "Made With Essential Oils" or "Made With Natural Ingredients". Claims like these do not state that the product is only made with the ingredient(s) specified. Such products may contain heavy proportions of synthetic fragrance oils and only contain a minute quantity of essential oil to simply be able to profess the "Made With Essential Oils" claim.

Essential oils, the pure essence of a plant, have been found to provide both psychological and physical benefits when used correctly and safely. The Essential Oil Profiles area details over 90 essential oils. Absolutes, CO2s and Hydrosols are also commonly utilized in aromatherapy. Although essential oils, CO2 extracts and absolutes are distilled in different manners, the term essential oil is sometimes used in writing as a blanket term to include CO2s and absolutes.

The essential oils are highly concentrated and should not be used directly. These oils can be blended together and this blend is called synergy. The synergy is more potent than the individual oils combined. To reduce the potency of these oils, you can dilute them by mixing them with carrier oils. Common carrier oils include sweet almond oil, apricot kernel oil and grape seed oil.

Benefits of Aromatherapy

1. The essential oils used in aromatherapy are the life force of the plants from which they have been extracted. These oils affect your mood. They enter through your olfactory system and affect the nervous system, thus improving mood and relaxing or energising you. For example, ylang ylang, chamomile and clary sage might help you beat anxiety and insomnia, while rosemary and geranium might be useful when your mood needs uplifting.

2. These oils can be massaged on your body, inhaled, added to your bath or sprayed in the air. When you take "Aromatherapy massage" with the essential oils, these oils are absorbed into the bloodstream via the skin. The constituents of essential oils can aid in health, beauty and hygiene conditions. Since essential oils are so powerful and concentrated, they should never be applied to the skin in their undiluted form. To apply essential oils to the skin, essential oils are typically diluted into a carrier such as a cold pressed vegetable oil, also known as a carrier oil.

3. Essential oils that are inhaled into the lungs offer both psychological and physical benefits. Not only does the aroma of the natural essential oil stimulate the brain to trigger a reaction, but when inhaled into the lungs, the natural constituents (naturally occurring chemicals) can supply therapeutic benefit. Diffusing eucalyptus

essential oil to help ease congestion is a prominent example.

4. Aromatherapy helps is in alleviating stress and speeding up healing.

5. These essential oils also have cosmetic properties and can be used in skin care and hair care products.

6. Many of these oils have known anti-viral, antifungal and antiseptic properties.

7. In addition to therapeutic benefit at the emotional and physical level, essential oils are helpful in other applications. These oils can be used in household and laundry cleaners.

8. Some oils act as a natural insect repellent and pesticide. You may recall using citronella candles during the summer to keep mosquitoes away. Citronella essential oil is the ingredient in the candles that is responsible for repelling the mosquitoes.

Essential oils differ in chemical composition from other herbal products because the distillation process only recovers the lighter phytomolecules. For this reason essential oils are rich in monoterpenes and sesquiterpenes, as well as other substances (esters, aromatic compounds, non-terpene hydrocarbons, some organic sulphides etc.).

Essential oils can be blended together to create appealing and complex aromas. Essential oils can also be blended for a specific therapeutic application. Essential oils that are carefully blended with a specific therapeutic purpose in mind may be referred to as an essential oil syngery. A synergistic essential oil blend is considered to be greater in total action than each oil working independently.

Aromatherapy Products

Today, with the great demand for essential oils and

aromatherapy products, there has been a wide range of products that claim to provide health benefits through aromatherapy which have arrived in the consumer market. Not all ready-made aromatherapy products labelled with the word "aromatherapy" are pure and natural. Products that contain artificial ingredients do not provide true aromatherapy benefits. At worst, they provide no benefit or are harmful. At best, they provide only a fraction of the benefit that natural products supply.

Buyers seeking true aromatherapy products must look at the ingredient label to ensure that the product does not contain fragrance oils or unpure (chemical) components. A general rule-of-thumb is to be wary of products that do not list their ingredients and those that do not boast of having pure essential oils (look for products that contain pure essential oils on their ingredient list and avoid those that have words like fragrance).

Essential oil diffusers are products that are expressly manufactured to help distribute the scent of the oils through the environment. These are usually especially made for aromatherapeutic purposes though some may be used to add fragrance to the air in a room.

Use of Other Complementary Natural Ingredients

In addition to essential oils, aromatherapy encourages the use of other complementary natural ingredients including cold pressed vegetable oils, jojoba (a liquid wax), hydrosols, herbs, milk powders, sea salts, sugars (an exfoliant), clays and muds. There are also a large variety of products that contain aromatherapies like candles, shampoo, lotions and soap.

Are Essential Oils Safe?

That depends. Essential oils can cause different reactions with different people. Many people might experience an allergic reaction or irritation from using essential oils. Also, essential oils found in clear bottles and chemical products like laundry detergents might not be so safe.

Light can harmfully alter the effectiveness of essential oils and many of the chemicals found in products like laundry detergents can ruin the effects of the essential oils.

Finally, keep in mind that not all aromatherapies have the same psychological effects on one group of people as on another.

Just add 3-6 aromatherapy essential oil drops into a shot of 6 ml vegetable oil bath foam. Dilute the mixture into water and stay in it for 20 minutes allowing the essential oil to infiltrate the skin while you enjoy the steam perfume. Choose an essential oil according to your mood: Rosemary or Sage oil in order to have a good start of your day; Lavender, Citronella or Melissa oil in order to calm and relax in the evening.

Massage

Add 3 drops of essential oils into 6 ml massage oil (approximately 1 small spoon) or into milky water. Choose an aromatherapy essential oil accordingly to your mood or condition: Camomile and Lavender oil after depilation; Savory, Ylang-Ylang and Cedar oil for a sensual massage.

Perfume

Aromatherapy essential oils are applied as individual perfumes or in combination. They can be used just for pleasure or in order to improve the effect of other aromatherapy applications. Add 2-6 drops into 6 ml of basic almond oil, Grape seed oil or Jojoba oil. For a pleasing perfume try a blend of Geranium and Mandarin oil. Men can add Vetiver, Cypress or Rosemary essential oil in their aftershave or tonic lotion.

Room Fragrance

Add 4-8 drops in a bowl of an aromatherapy essential oil burner. Fill it with water and put it over a candle. It is the ideal natural way to kill every smell. Sage, Laurel and Eucalyptus are used to clean microbes in the air, while Lemon, Mandarin, Orange and Pennyroyal essential oils are used to clean room air from tobacco smoke and make a pleasant atmosphere.

Hair

Essential oils invigorate the scalp and take care of hair follicles contributing to better hair health and appearance. Camomile and Lavender oil are suitable for very dry and weathered hair. Add 3 drops into 6 ml hot massage oil and lightly rub your head. Then after giving your head a rinse with a shampoo, muffle your head with a towel for 20 minutes and. You can also add the aromatherapy essential oil of your choice to the conditioner or to the final rinse. For grassy hair try Camomile, Cedar wood, Geranium or Mandarin essential oil. Cedar wood, Rosemary and Laurel oils are used for hair lose (for men and women), while Rosemary and Cypress are appropriate as a hair tonic.

Facial and Skin Care

Aromatherapy essential oils help sebaceous glands to function properly improving the whole skin health. Add 2 essential oils drops every 6 ml of cleansing cream, tonic lotion or milky water and create your unique cosmetics. You can make mixtures that can last for weeks, but remember that essential oil's attributes are more effective when the blend is fresh.

Babies and Children Care

Aromatherapy essential oils are very wholesome and beneficial for babies and children as far as they are used carefully. Before applying them to their sensitive skin, essential oils should be diluted into cleansing cream or water. For babies, it is better to add only 1 drop of essential oils into 10 ml of cream. Respectively, add 1 drop for every 6 ml of cream, lotion or milky water for children (half of the adult's dose). The children's deep sleep can be facilitated by Lavender essential oil, while Mandarin calms and soothes.

9

Bachflower Therapy

What is Bach Flower Therapy?

Bach flower therapy is a form of energy medicine and Bach flower essences (remedies) form a part of alternative medicine. They comprise a therapeutic system that uses dilutions of flower essences to balance physical and emotional disturbances.

Bach flower therapy brings together two very important principles in the art of human healing. The first is that the source for chronic disorders, even long term physical states, is rooted in states of disorder in the human psyche (conflicts, shocks, fears, chronic anger, jealousy, etc.).

Bach flower essences (remedies) are similar to homeopathy in many respects. Bach flower essences are not dependent on the theory of successive dilutions, and are not based on the homeopathy's defining principle the 'Law of Similars' ('Like cures like'). Another difference between homoeopathy and Bach flower remedies are the methods used to produce them.

Dr. Edward Bach

Bach flower therapy is named after Dr. Edward Bach, whose research led to its development in England in the 1930's. Bach flower therapy has now been in use for over 60 years.

In the world of flowers Dr. Bach found resonances of the conditions he found in his patients. He believed the right essence can help to bring back the patient to a positive, happy condition. Dr. Bach distilled the essence of certain flowers, and chose the right ones for the state of being of a patient.

Dr. Bach knew that the human being is more than a physical body. The human being incorporates a body of life energy, a body of sensitivity and feelings, and a spiritual body. Flower essences are energetic imprints of the life force of plants. Dr Bach believed that the flower essences interact with the subtle bodies and so can help people with physical illness by addressing the emotional responses to their illness.

Since life all around us demonstrates an almost limitless capacity to recover and heal, if a condition of illness is not resolving then it stands to reason that something is preventing it from doing so. In the case of human emotionally conditioned states, if the psychic disturbance can be rebalanced then there must necessarily by a natural resurgence in health.

This brings us to the second principle which is essential to this particular art of healing - the Flower Therapy. Bach felt that the answer to problems of living must be found in the realm of the living.

Historically and until recently, the vast majority of medicinal substances were found in the plant realm and Dr Bach felt that nature provides the best solutions to one's own problems, and this includes human illness.

With a background in homoeopathy and familiarity with homoeopathic "pictures" of many plants and flowers, coupled with his own delicate insight into the qualities of individual plants, Bach was able to isolate 38 flowers for essential characteristics which match what Bach held to be the full spectrum of human emotional disorders. Each of the flowers he decided on relates to a particular emotional dysfunction, whether it is fear, mistrust, despair, anger, etc. All this came to be popularly known as Bach flower therapy.

The production of Bach flower essences is handled in two ways, called 'potentisation': the sun method and the boiling method, both invented by Dr. Bach.

Bach Flower Remedy

A Bach flower "remedy" consists of water that has been patterned with the energetic vibrations of one of 38 different flowers. The remedy is added to a cup of water (or other beverage) four times a day. Like other energetic healing modalities, this treatment seeks to create balance in areas of energetic disruption. Bach flower treatment specifically addresses the emotional body of the energy system. Its purpose is to restore emotional harmony.

All negative emotions can be addressed with Bach flower therapy. Unlike psychotropic medications (i.e. medicines that treat depression, anxiety or psychosis), Bach flowers treat specific shades of emotion, like anger, fear guilt, inferiority complex, lack of confidence, negative expectancy, envy, jealousy etc. by flooding the consciousness with positive feelings.

In Bach flower therapy, "disturbed" feelings, moods, attitudes are taken as base for the selection of medicine. Bach found these "imbalances" in the personality as the "core element of disease". Bach flower therapy is thus all about correcting these imbalances.

Bach flower remedies are used individually and along with other remedies. The most popular remedy is rescue remedy; this remedy is the combination of equal amounts of rock rose, impatiens, clematis, star of Bethlehem and cherry plum remedies. Rescue remedy is used for treating stress, anxiety and panic attacks. Rescue cream is applied externally for minor skin problems such as burns and itches.

There are 38 original Bach remedies plus 'Rescue Remedy', each prescribed for certain mental and emotional problems.

They form a complete therapeutic system. Practitioners treat every variety of human emotional imbalance with the 38 Bach flower essences.

Differences between Bach Flower Therapy and Traditional Medical Therapy

There are important differences between Bach flower therapy and traditional medical therapy. Bach flowers are not medicinal. They can be taken along with any food, herb, health product or medicine without causing any interaction. In this way, they are most similar to water. Bach flowers treat the unhealthy emotional tendency, meaning that when the disturbing emotion is no longer active, flower treatment is stopped. One does not continue treatment in such a case, because the flower does not act preventatively like vitamins or medicine. Rather, it operates more like a process that undoes a knot (in the energetic flow). Once the knot is undone, there is no further need to keep undoing it!

The Safety and Effectiveness of Bach Flowers

Bach flowers can be taken safely by infants, pregnant or nursing women, the elderly, and even those who have flower allergies. Again, just as water itself cannot harm this population, Bach flowers cannot cause negative reactions. Indeed, thinking of Bach flower remedies as being a collection of harmonious water crystals is really the most accurate way to conceptualise them.

However, these remedies are preserved with a small amount of brandy. Those that are allergic to brandy or who cannot take it for other reasons, can still utilise Bach flower therapy. Remedies need not be taken internally - they can be put directly on pulse points on the skin.

Psychotropic medications have been subjected to extensive therapeutic trials before being put on the market. As a result, their specific actions and negative side effects are clearly defined, as are some of their underlying mechanisms. Nonetheless, even medicines are not completely understood in the effects they have on the human body (and even less so, for many of those currently being used on children). In contrast, only a small number of clinical trials have been published on Bach Flower Treatment in North America. However, these tentatively point to a positive effect on stress and mood.

When one decides to experiment with Bach flower therapy, one should keep in mind that no treatment of any kind works equally well for everyone. Therefore, while many people experience excellent results with Bach therapy, others do not notice any effect at all. A fair trial, however, should last weeks or months (depending on the therapist's recommendation), rather than a couple of days.

Bach flower therapy is gentle and subtle, so that improvements tend to happen gradually and almost imperceptibly. It can be helpful to keep a brief written record of weekly mood descriptions, in order to track improvements and changes.

Bach flower therapy can be used as a self-help tool by anyone to help soothe daily irritability, moodiness and stress of all kinds. However, when problems are deeper, repetitive, or chronic, psychological counselling may be more appropriate.

Often, flower remedies can be used during the counselling process as a form of support between sessions or as a way of facilitating the psychological work itself.

The Twelve Healers

Dr Bach's discovery of the first flower essences became known as the twelve healers; these flowers are:

1. Impatiens – the time flower
2. Mimulus – the bravery flower
3. Clematis – the reality flower
4. Agrimony – the honesty flower
5. Chicory – the motherliness flower

6. Vervain – the enthusiasm flower
7. Centaury – the service flower
8. Cerato – the intuition flower
9. Sceleranthus – the balance flower
10. Water Violet – the communication flower
11. Gentian – the belief flower
12. Rock Rose – the liberation flower.

Dr. Bach discovered additional flower remedies which included the Four Helpers – Gorse, Oak, Heather and Rock Water; however, perhaps his most famous Bach flower remedy which is used worldwide today is the first-aid remedy, Rescue, a combination of the flower essences Impatiens, Star of Bethlehem, Cherry Plum, Rock Rose and Clematis. The Bach Rescue Remedy is extremely useful for the treatment of stress, shock and anxiety.

Further study of the Bach flower essences and therapy is needed to fully understand and use the Bach flower remedies devised by Dr. Edward Bach; however, not only can the flower remedies be used for humans but Bach flower remedies are a useful tool in treating animals too.

❖❖❖

10

Chiropractic

What is Chiropractic?

Chiropractic is generally considered to be a complementary and alternative medicine. Chiropractic medicine operates on the theory that the improper alignment of the vertebrae (there are twenty-four verterbrae that make up the spinal column) and the spinal cord they protect is the cause of diseases and disorders.

Chiropractic is a health care approach and profession that emphasizes diagnosis, treatment and prevention of mechanical disorders of the musculoskeletal system, especially the spine, under the hypothesis that these disorders affect general health via the nervous system. For patients with uncomplicated, acute low back pain, chiropractic has also been found to be effective.

Treatment Procedure

Chiropractors apply pressure in a specific manner to allow the vertebrae in the spinal column to realign themselves. But most chiropractors do more than manipulating the spinal column. They are whole body healers by paying attention to factors such as nutrition, stress management, etc.

The main treatment involves manual therapy including manipulation of the spine, other joints, and soft tissue; treatment also includes exercises and health and lifestyle counselling. Chiropractors help in dealing with low back pain, sciatica, neck pain, and other syndromes related to the spine. If you have back pain, it's reasonable to make a chiropractor's office your first stop.

It is estimated that more people see chiropractors for back problems than for all other ailments combined.

Benefit of Chiropractic

Chiropractic spinal manipulation has been recognised by the health officials worldwide as an effective therapy for acute low-back pain. Chiropractic treatment has been found to be more beneficial to patients with persistent back and neck complaints than other forms of manipulation.

Research in Great Britain found chiropractic to provide worthwhile, long-term benefits for patients with low back pain in comparison to hospital outpatient management. This study also found chiropractic benefits to persist for a three-year period, indicating long-term benefits.

A cost comparison study of back-related injuries showed the number of work days lost for patients treated with chiropractic to be nearly ten times less than that of patients treated under medical care.

Traditional versus Chiropractic

Traditional chiropractic therapy relies on spinal mani-pulation to correct misaligned vertebrae, which may be responsible for problems anywhere along the spine. According to practitioners, misalignment of the verte-brae in the spine can cause the joints to press on the spinal nerves, leading to direct pain in the back and possibly "referred" pain in other parts of the body. By helping restore motion to poorly functioning vertebrae, chiropractic therapy diminishes the accompanying pain and muscle spasm.

Chiropractic is a harmless therapy and, if it does not help you, you can always go to see an orthopedist. In fact, English orthopedists are also trained to manipulate the spine unlike their American counterparts.

The straight chiropractors, who confine their practice to dealing with the bony structures of the body, can provide a great deal of relief and a healing touch for many musculoskeletal problems. They are trained to recognise what they should treat and what they should not treat.

Ailments Curable by Chiropractic

Chiropractic is effectively used for the following:

1. Effectiveness of Chiropractic
2. Addiction
3. Asthma
4. Autonomic Nervous System
5. Back Pain
6. Back & Neck Problems
7. Bedwetting
8. Cancer
9. Colic
10. Ear Infections
11. Glaucoma
12. Migraines
13. Premenstrual Syndrome

Importance of Maintaining Good Posture

One of the most common reasons for health problems that I see in my office is faulty posture. Having poor posture will almost guarantee that you'll have chiropractic structural problems. But luckily, if you get proper chiropractic spinal and extremity adjustments and are put on a postural rehabilitation program, postural faults will not plague you.

What constitutes good posture?

If you drop a line down from your head to your feet it should pass directly through the following:

1. Ear canal
2. Shoulder joint

3. Hip joint
4. Knee joint
5. Ankle joint

Effects of Poor Posture

The immediate effect of having poor posture is that you'll start to develop abnormal pains in your body. These are pains that you have no idea why they're there. You'll begin to notice that you'll have upper neck, back and low back pain. You may even develop foot, knee and hip pain.

How to Correct Poor Posture?

Step 1: Make sure that you are analysed by a competent chiropractic physician (preferably one who focuses on postural alignment and is also very familiar with Applied Kinesiology or Muscle Response Testing.).

Step 2: Remove structural interferences in all affected joints. Chiropractors term these interferences "subluxations". These subluxations interfere with your joint's normal motion and restricted motion is the first step toward postural distortions.

Step 3: Focus on retraining the surrounding stabilising muscles. This is most important to a lasting postural correction. Along with making sure the surrounding muscles are "firing at optimal" your chiropractor should then make sure all the surrounding muscles move together in a synchronous pattern. When the muscles move synchronously you decrease the wear and tear on the joint.

Step 4: Focus on general postural enhancing exercises. There are specific exercises that will help you to regain proper posture. Some include: chin-tuck, abdominal bracing and pelvic rocking.

11

Chromotherapy

History of Chromotherapy

The use of colour as a therapy is a truly holistic, non-invasive and powerful therapy which dates back thousands of years; evidence of this can be found in ancient texts from India, China and Egypt.

The use of colour therapy has a long history. The ancient Egyptians and Greeks built healing temples of light and colour. In India and China, colour carried a greater impact, and it remains an integral part in ayurvedic medicine. In US and Europe, the therapeutic use of colour was developed in the second half of the 19th century.

What is Chromotherapy?

Colour is simply light of varying wavelengths and, as such, is a form of energy that is used in Colour Therapy or Chromotherapy. Colour energy can be the catalyst for our healing process and encourages normal and healthy workings of the body.

Chromotherapy, sometimes called colour therapy or colourology, is an alternative medicine method. It is claimed that a therapist trained in chromotherapy can use colour and light to balance energy wherever a person's body is lacking, be it physical, emotional, spiritual or mental. Of course it should not be confused with Light Therapy, which has been proven to relieve things like major depressive disorder.

Colour therapy is another important component of naturopathy. It is used for giving relief to physical and psychological disorders. Every colour will have an emotional effect on your nerves. Different colours have different properties.

Colour theory offers a way to enhance nearly every aspect of our lives - improving our moods and stimu-lating our minds, increasing our effectiveness at work and in society, and creating better physical and mental health.

Colour therapy can be used for any problem, whether physical, mental, emotional or spiritual for specific problems as well as an over all relaxation therapy. Colour therapy can be used safely and effectively - either alone or alongside any other therapy, whether complementary or orthodox medicine - for adults, children, babies and non-human animals alike.

Colour therapy should not be something you just go to a therapist to 'have done to you'. Colour is everywhere and should be utilised as part of our everyday life. A professional colour therapist can explain and advise you on how you can use colour at home for health and well-being.

Application of Colour for Healing

Colour is simply light of different wavelengths, and each colour has its own specific wavelength and vibration. These wavelengths resonate with energies in different areas of the body.

As we absorb colour energy not only through the eyes but also through the skin and the electro magnetic field or aura, colour therapy can be used on the body in a number of different ways.

When performing chromotherapy, colour and light are applied to specific areas and acupoints on the body. Because colours get associated with both positive and negative effects in colour therapy, specific colours and accurate amounts of colour are deemed to be critical in healing.

Scientists have studied the effects of colour on our mood, health and way of thinking over the years. Colours are visible light of certain wavelengths. It enters our bodies, stimulates the pituitary and pineal glands, affects certain hormones and in turn our physiological process is varied. This explains why colours have been found to have direct influence on our mind, thoughts, moods and behaviour.

Understanding Yourself with Colour

Some of us love yellow, some of us hate orange. We all have our colour preferences.

There is a reason for these colour preferences which can be explained thus:

Either by life experiences involving that colour - a negative life experience will make us dislike a certain colour; a positive life experience involving a particular colour will, of course, make us feel drawn to that colour.

Or an aversion to a colour can indicate an imbalance in that particular area of the body.

Being aware of these preferences can tell us a great deal about ourselves and help us to address sometimes, very deep seated emotional issues, character traits etc.

Colour can be incredibly enlightening and transforming.

Pink and green convey vitality, red symbolises justice, white represents pureness and black denotes a sense of awe, grandeur and depth. No colour is universally is useful in all cultures for the maintenance of internal harmony within individuals and external harmony between them and nature.

Studies have revealed that people who are very fond of mauve, red, violet, blue and purple or often use these colours in their daily life are very sympathetic in nature. They always aim to have a successful relationship after marriage. They like their husband / wife to hold a topmost position and try to help them in their day-to-day work. They are sacrificing kind of people in nature.

People who love black colour feel lonely even in a huge crowd. Their thinking is philosophical and they love to stay alone. But if loneliness extends then people should avoid using this colour and instead they should use bright colours.

People, who prefer blue, are always confident and are soft hearted. They always wait for the right scope to avail. Blue is so fine so very sublime so ever beautifully blue.

Red is a vibrant colour. People who love red are stubborn in nature. They love to fight the situation and do anything to make it in their way. But they denote simplicity. They don't like criticism or backbiting. Red can be frightful even delightful but always surprisingly red.

People attracted to pastel shades are the one who don't like changes frequently. They are very hardworking and dedicated towards their work. They get success in their life all of a sudden.

Yellow is gracious, warm and vivacious ever expansively yellow.

Green is suitable so multitudable so ever wonderfully green Orange at least is a veritable feast ever so edible orange.

Colour also indicates cardinal directions, seasons, the cyclical passage of time, and the internal organs of the human body. Colour is regarded as a manifestation of cosmic energy - vitality that can also shape an individuals personal energy and therefore, their destiny. Adding a new colour to an environment can stimulate a positive or negative response.

Association of Colours with Elements

Five elements of nature, i.e., Air, Fire, Earth, Water and Space, are responsible for generating positive and negative energies. These five elements are not physical substances but powers or essences describing all matter and all attributes. These elements are also associated with colours, seasons, directions and organs. For example, the elements.

'Fire' is associated with red, summer, the south, the heart.

'Earth' positioned at the center, stands for yellow, oranges, or brown, mid-autumn, etc. and the liver.

'Air' is blue autumn, north and the lungs and gall bladder it gets), winter, the west, and the kidneys.

'Space' is shapeless, colourless and has north-east direction effects mind and cells.

A rainbow sighted in the east indicates fine weather, while to the west it means rain. A red sky in the morning will foretell an afternoon shower, while a red sky at night will mean a clear sky. A halo around the moon indicates wind.

Benefits of Colour Therapy

1. Colours affect various domains of our life - world, food, clothing, the living place, transportation, education and recreation. A wise arrangement of colours will help to increase your happiness, enhance your wealth, and foster your marital harmony.
2. Colour inspires emotion. Colour structures our behaviour.
3. All permutations, from cosmic to atomic, resound in us and the force that links us with colour is energy or cosmic breath. Energy is the non-biological self, i.e., our spirit, our psyche, our essence. Without energy, we are merely flesh and bones. Energy is the breath essential to maintaining physical, environmental and emotional balance. In a sense, it is destiny, a blueprint of our personality, talent and life course.

4. Colour also can harmonise and balance our energy, and thus improve our life and destiny. For any form known to exist, it must possess colour and we know that out of the void of the universe come all things. Harmony and balance are desirable in our physical and emotional makeup and in our environment. Out of the balance and harmonising of positive and negative forces arises energy - the most essential feature of life and life and human energy is greatly affected by colour.
5. Colours, full of life force (energy) - green, blue, bluish-purple, reddish-purple - stimulate the brain, providing access to energy. Such colours help them to work hard and concentrate. This light energy affects all living cells (as we all know, without light all living things are affected). Used in the right way, these different frequencies of light, i.e. colour, can have a profound and healing effect on all creation, human or otherwise. It is a well known scientific fact that everything has a vibration, that is to say that all things have their own vibration/frequency, and that includes us!
6. From ancient times to the present, the colours of nature have provided a calming and invigorating stimulus to our bodies and minds, enhancing our emotions, speech and nervous system, the reds, blues, greens, yellows and whites of trees, flowers, and earth help to inspire and regenerate our energy.
7. All colours of nature are highly evocative. Today, life is complicated and confusing, and our minds can become unsettled and weighed down by work, daily activities and struggles. So we take vacations each year to rest and travel, to go to the mountains or the seashore to regenerate ourselves. We need to see colours that we do not normally see often, to bring balance to our minds and bodies and to stimulate our energy. This colourful change is, in a sense, enjoyment.

8. In our daily life, colour has a huge role to play. It can heal us from many diseases or psychological disorders. Colours can enhance our personality or even can rain fortunes on a person. For example if you see blue colour it gives soothing and calming effect on your nerves. When you see yellow colour it stimulates your intelligence. Colour therapy will restore your mental balances and improve the healing process in your body.
9. Using of alternate colours will be beneficial for everyone in spite of using the same one frequently. Colours can bring good fortune to anyone's life if they are being correctly used in daily life. People should practise the perfect way to influence these colours in their daily life whether for physical ailment or for their psychological disorders as well. Thus we find that using right colours may make one successful in life and bring prosperity to him when he uses the colours in the correct way.
10. Colours can treat one from asthma to yellow fever.
11. In allergy one can increase the use of indigo and soft orange, or a person suffering from typhoid can use more amount of green to cure it. Likewise colours can treat several diseases.

Colour therapy is a totally holistic and non-invasive therapy for us all - adults, children, babies and animals. All we need to do is to heighten our awareness of the energy of colour and it can transform our lives.

Colour should be a part of our everyday life, not just something we experience for an hour or two with a therapist. Colour is all around us everywhere. This wonderful planet does not contain all the beautiful colours of the rainbow without reason. Nature and its colours are not simply here by chance, everything in nature is here for a purpose. Colour is no exception.

The capacity for health and well being is within us all - let colour therapy help you to fulfil your potential.

Common Methods of Treatment

As with any therapy, each therapist may have his or her own 'style'. However, a number of common methods used are:

1. The placing of colour silks on the body
2. The directing of coloured light on to the body (A light box is the most common form of directing colour to the body using coloured filters)
3. Solarised water
4. Meditation with colour
5. Colour breathing

Colour choices can indicate where there may be an imbalance of colour which can highlight a potential problem; whether emotional, physical, mental or spiritual, and also give indications of personality issues which may need to be addressed.

The emotional, physical, mental and spiritual aspects make up the whole person, and really one cannot be isolated from the other.

A professionally qualified colour therapy practitioner will help you to understand your colour preferences, and indeed your need for a certain colour or colours. Your colour preferences can tell a professional colour therapist a good deal about you.

Colours describe emotional properties. We feel blue or green with anyone; we associate red with shyness; we describe someone as "a yellow-coward".

The properties of colour are both emotional and physical. The direct impact of colour on our existence is easy to understand. Some colours make us happy, other colours make us sink into gloom, and some others help to relax, distract or energise us.

Colour is a manifestation of light and energy. A good colour can depend on your mood of the day. If you select a colour that harmonises with your energy then you will flourish. If the colour clashes with your mood, that colour will irritate you. Whatever we look upon and see through our eyes will, through our optic nerve, send sensory signals to our body, to react to what our eyes see. So the colours of everything our eyes come in contact with will influence our temperament, physical movements, language and thoughts - in short, our lives.

Tools for Applying Colours

Some of the tools used for applying colors are gemstones, candles, wands, prisms, coloured fabrics, bath treatments, and coloured glasses or lenses.

Therapeutic colour can be administered in a number of ways, but is often combined with hydrotherapy and aromatherapy in an attempt to heighten the therapeutic effect.

Enhance Your Life with Colour

Have you taken inventory of your closet lately? You may be in a fashion rut and need to introduce some new articles of clothing into your wardrobe with different colours that will best reflect your mood swings. Wearing the wrong colour can make you feel out of sorts with yourself.

1. Wearing Green - Nurturing and Earthy

Green is considered to be one of the most healing among all the colours.

Because green is the colour of trees and grasses it is a wonderful colour choice to wear anytime you are wanting to feel more in-tune with nature. Green represents the Spring season and new growth. Choose this colour to wear whenever you are embarking on something new or wish to turn over a new leaf.

Hug a Tree

Embrace Mother Nature

2. Wearing Blue - Serenity and Calm

Wearing blue helps create a place of calm and serenity.

Wearing ocean hues of blue is especially calming. Indigo or darker blues can offer more of a comfort zone feeling, almost as if you are sinking into a pool of warm water. Blues in general remind me of a favorite pair of well-worn denim jeans - now that's simply relaxing.

Creating a Serene Sacred Space

Ways to Calm an Anxious Spirit

3. Wearing Gray or Black - Invisibility and Blending In

Wearing grays and blacks can be depressive.

Let's face it, black and gray are fashion basics. We all have the basic black suit or black dress slacks that are a must wear for a number of different social settings. Aside from the slinky spaghetti strapped number you have hanging in the back of the closet, you likely choose to wear black because you prefer to blend in and not make any statement. Wearing black will allow you to keep a low-profile in social settings if that is your intention. Don't wear black if you want to stand out amidst a crowd. Most folks don't even bother to wear black at funerals anymore, it's just too sad to wear dreary and dark colours.

Symptoms of Depression

4. Wearing Orange - Energetic and Creative

Orange urges you to get out into the world and create something grand!

Orange is a very high energy colour. Its creativity juices are extremely intoxicating and sweet tasting. Wearing orange is fun and can make you feel quite playful. Artists love dabbling with orange hues. Orange screams with sexual energy too, not surprising since orange is associated with the sacral chakra.

Because of its highly-charged intensity some people cannot comfortably wear this colour. Adorning yourself with an orange accent piece can add a hint of playfulness. Beware, if you need to complete a mundane project avoid wearing orange as it might interfere with the stick-to-it-ness required to stay on task.

Sacral Chakra

Art Therapy

5. Wearing Pink - Open Heart

Wearing pink conveys compassion and an open heart.

Most people associate pink with babies, little girls, and feminine energies. But more than feeling feminine, wearing pink conveys compassion and an open heart. When people are wearing pink, whether they are male or female, they appear approachable and capable of loving others. If you want to feel heart-connected reach for that pastel pink sweater from your closet to wear. And if pastel colours don't suit you try on something in bright fuchsia. You'll feel pretty in pink.

Rose Quartz Meditation

Language of Love

6. Wearing Purple - Unique and Special

Wearing purple shows others that you want to be noticed.

Purple is seldom worn as a neutral color. Purple is the wrong colour choice to make if you are wanting to blend in among others as you go about your business. The colour purple, especially shades of violet, will definitely make a statement. Wearing purple shows others that you want to be noticed. If it is your desire to feel special and unique then purple is the right colour choice. If you would like to send a message out into the world that you're one of a kind and that you could care less about conformity, then wear purple.

You Are the Colours You Choose

Colour Your Life

7. Wearing Red - Powerful and Confident

Red can really pack a punch when needed.

Red is a very powerful colour. Wear red whenever you feel a need to portray confidence or would like to boost your self esteem. However, be aware that wearing too much red can make a person come off a little too intimidating to others who may lack self confidence in themselves. Visualising the colour red can help ground your energies so anyone who has "flighty" tendencies will benefit from wearing red to serve as a reminder to ground themselves throughout the day.

Visualising the Colour Red

Root Chakra

8. Wearing White - Fresh Outlook - New Beginnings

Wearing white will help reduce any nagging feelings of disappointment or drudge.

White represents cleansing and new beginnings. Putting on a white blouse feels like being given an opportunity to start the day with a clean slate. Wearing a white garment, as long as it hasn't taken on any discolouration from too much laundering, can offer a fresh and bright outlook. Be sure to get rid of any dingy white clothes often, replacing them with brighter whites.

White Light

New Moon Ritual

9. Wearing Yellow - Cheerful and Happy

Yellow is the perfect colour to wear whenever your spirits needs an uplift.

Yellow carries the same healing qualities associated with the sun. It offers warmth, optimism, and light. All shades of yellows and golds will cheer you up and help make you feel happier. Wearing yellow out into the world makes an affirmation statement. For certain, yellow is a perky colour!

Choosing Happiness

Affirmations

❖❖❖

12

Homoeopathy

What is Homoeopathy?

Homoeopathy is a therapeutic method of medicine in which very dilute doses of natural active substances (plant, animal, or mineral origins) are administered to a patient to treat symptoms that would be induced in a healthy individual by ingestion of that same substance.

Conventional medicine attempts to restore health by killing invading organisms, replacing hormones or enzymes, or interfering with disease processes. Calcium blockers are an example. Homoeopathy is an approach to health that is quite different from methods that are seen in the pharmacy everyday. Homoeopathy stimulates the body's own defences to correct illness and allow symptoms to dissipate. The minute dose of drug substance used in homoeopathy does not cause any of the side effects that have become such a problem for the physician, pharmacist and patient.

History of Homoeopathy

Homoeopathy was known and employed five hundred years before the birth of Christ by the Greek physician Hippocrates. This dosage-dependent, contradictory action of medically active substances was not to become universally known until it was rediscovered by Samuel Hahnemann, M.D., a German physician, in1796.

Dr. Hahnemann, distressed by the barbaric medical methods of his day, like bleeding, purging, and the use of leeches, chose to leave the practice of medicine and supported his family by translating medical, scientific and botanical books. It was during this period that he uncovered the ancient 'Principle of Similars'.

Hahnemann's first application of this newly-found principle was his observation of the toxicologic effects of cinchona bark, which was then being used to treat malaria. The bark often produced attacks of fever very much like the malaria fever. When tiny doses of the homoeopathic cinchona were administered to the malaria-infected patients, the malaria fevers were reduced. From his own observations, Hahnemann deduced that infinitesimal doses of medicinal substances were capable of curing symptoms similar to those which they could produce. He named his discovery 'The Principle of Similars'. After his discovery, he spent the rest of his years developing and cataloguing the relationship between disease and conditions (symptoms) and the toxic effects of natural, medically-active substances.

Proving

Administration of crude quantities of these substances to a healthy individual with the intention of developing a symptom picture is called a 'proving'. Clinically, an individual who has a disease displays a certain group of symptoms, which can be identified with the same symptom-complex that has been developed and catalogued in the health volunteer proving group. Clinically, the substance that produces the same symptom complex during the proving which the patient is currently exhibiting in his illness is the remedy prescribed by the physician.

Principle of Similars

The most common example offered to explain this Principle of Similars is Ipecac. A large dose of Ipecac is given to a healthy individual to induce vomiting. However, a patient suffering from nausea and vomiting improves when a homoeopathic dose of Ipecac is administered.

The Principle of Similars of homoeopathy may be summarised as:

a. Every pharmacologically active substance produces symptoms in a healthy, sensitive individual which are characteristic of that substance.
b. Each disease has a characteristic set of symptoms.
c. An illness can be cured by administering to a patient a small, homoeopathically prepared dose of the same substance which, during a proving, produced symptoms similar to the illness in healthy individuals.

Wide Use of Homoeopathic Products

Homoeopathic medicines are different from herbal products. In addition to conventional drugs, homoeopathic drug products are the only other form of official and regulated medicine in many countries. Homoeopathic medicines are now receiving a much higher level of consumer interest. As patients explore alternative medical methods, pharmacists are asked to comment about natural and homoeopathic drug products. They are also asked common questions about effectiveness, reliability, possible interactions with other medications, or how they are regulated or approved.

Today there are over 2,000 substances catalogued that describe symptom pictures of the most common conditions like allergies, colds, flu and bruises.

Homoeopathy is truly a safer medicine - because it has no harmful side effects!

Energy Medicine

Homoeopathic medicine, by a special process of attenuation or dilution, is able to use the vital energy from any substance at all - from plants to animals, to metals to minerals, to the sun and moon and even to music.

In homoeopathy we then look at the differing characteristics from these substances. For example plants have different likes and dislikes, some like it hot, some like it shady or damp. This helps to make them flower seed and survive as a species. Plants are very sensitive and feel a lot - so do plant people. Many people have heard of Arnica, the flower which grows at the foot of a mountain. It is told to be very good for bruises and accident trauma i.e. falling down a mountain! Nature is kind and supplies us with all our needs.

Why Energy Medicine?

When we have physical, mental or emotional symptoms our vitality is low and has allowed illness to come in - "the defences are down". This is because we are out of balance or even suffering on an emotional (or energetic) level. This energy depletion needs energy to stimulate a return to health. How often do you hear people say they have no energy or they are depressed?

It is very difficult to explain the feeling experienced after a good remedy. People are often on an energy high at first and then settle down to a level where they can manage their lives to their best advantage. The best way to experience this is to try homoeopathy! Even if you feel there is nothing wrong with you can benefit from it to maintain good health.

Although no one knows precisely how homoeopathic medicines initiate the healing process, there is over 200 years of experience by hundreds of thousands of clinicians and tens of millions of patients that these medicines they have powerful effects. One cannot help but sense and anticipate the veritable treasure-trove of knowledge that further research in homoeopathy and nanopharmacology will bring in this new millennium.

13

Magneto Therapy

Magnetic field therapy diagnoses and treats both physical and emotional pain. It relieves symptoms and retards the cycle of new disease. Magneto therapy itself does not cure but it can provide the magnetic conditions in which the body's healing forces operate at their optimum level. Magnetism stimulates the body to heal itself.

What is Magneto Therapy?

Magnets and electromagnetic therapy devices are now being used to eliminate pain, facilitate healing of broken bones, and counter the effects of stress. Magnet therapy, magnetic therapy, magneto therapy or magno therapy is a complementary and alternative medicine practice involving the use of static magnetic fields.

Magneto therapy is used as complementary or supplementary to another system of medicine as and when needed. It has proved beneficial in certain diseases, especially in rheumatic and muscular aches and pains, as it has the power of draining pains out of the body.

Magneto therapy is all about using magnets to treat various kind of ailments. Magneto therapy is a system of treating patients with the use of magnets. Not only the magnet but even magnetised water has been found to have very favourably acted on human diseases and has worked as a beneficial medicine in many cases.

A magnet has many healing properties. It not only attracts iron but also attracts all martial humors that are in the human system of blood; phlegm, black bile and yellow bile, of which the body in ancient medicine was thought to be composed. The magnet is useful in internal and external diseases. This alternative treatment benefits from the important interrelationship between electromagnetic energy and the human body.

History of Magneto Therapy

For thousands of years Chinese, Egyptians, Chaldeans, Arabs, Greeks, Romans and Indians have used magnets to heal. According to legend, about 2,500 years ago, a shepherd named Magnes found mineral stones sticking to the metal nails in his sandals. That mineral received the name magnetite.

History is rife with evidences of the use of magnet therapy from ancient times.

The healing power of magnets is mentioned even in *Atharvaveda* which was written centuries back in India.

In 2000 B.C., magnetic stones are mentioned in the oldest medical textbook ever discovered, the *Yellow Emperor's Classic of Internal Medicine.*

In the 4th century B.C., the philosopher Aristotle was fascinated by magnets. And near the turn of the millennium Cleopatra, the beautiful Egyptian queen, is reported to have worn a magnet on her forehead. In the same century, Martel, a French doctor, used magnets to heal hand and feet's pain.

In the 6th century, Alexandre de Tralles cured joint's pain with magnets. Hall Abbas, an Arab doctor, used it to treat spasms and feet's pain.

In the 16th century, Paracelsus, the European doctor, used magnets for inflammation. He was a brilliant thinker and a pioneer for many future magnet healers.

In the 17th century, the court physician to Elizabeth I, William Gilbert, used "lodestones" (magnets) to heal bleeding and for its astringent's properties.

In the 18th century, the French Royal Society of Medicine concluded that magnets are antispasmodic, relieve strong pains and "can neither be ignored nor contested". The German doctor Mesmer was a famous, but controversial magnet healer. It's questionable whether he did more to advance or hinder magnet therapy. He was a flamboyant showman and public relations self-promoter. Patients flocked to him and this gave magnet therapy much publicity, for better or for worse.

In the 19th century, Doctor Magiorani and Charcot used it sucessfully too.

In 1925, a french doctor, Durville, wrote a book about magnetotherapy, giving instructions to cure dozen of ailments with magnets.

In 1976, in Boston (U.S.A.), the first International Conference on Biomagnetism was held.

In 1991, in Munster, Germany, the eighth International Conference on Biomagnetism featured 240 presentations and attracted 400 participants. Magnetic therapy had arrived.

In 1983, one of the greatest discoveries ever in magnetics was announced. Rare earth neodymium biomagnets were invented which are 700 per cent as powerful as the older ceramic magnets. The neodymium biomagnets hold their charge indefinitely, with no significant loss of power after 10 years. At first, their cost was prohibitive, but now they are very economical.

The legends of Aristotle and Cleopatra have now been tested by 21st century scientific studies which results will amaze you.

Today magnet therapy is seeing a resurgence in use, and is an officially approved therapy in over 45 countries worldwide. In the history of medical science for pain relief, there has been no greater discovery than biomagnet therapy. And it is growing at a phenomenal pace.

Until recently, although the health improving potential of magnet therapy was well documented, scientific explanation of magnetic action was not available. Dedicated researchers and the introduction of the space age have contributed greatly to the understanding of the physiology of magnetism in health and healing.

Establishment of Magnetic Field Therapy

The world is surrounded by magnetic fields: some generated by the earth's magnetism, others generated by solar storms and changes in weather. Magnetic fields are also created by electrical devices. Even the human body produces a subtle magnetic fields generated by chemical reaction within cells and ionic currents of the nervous system. Recently, scientists discovered that external magnetic fields affect the body's functioning in both positive and negative ways. The observation of this led to the establishment of the magnetic field therapy.

All magnets have two poles, one positive and one negative. In 1974 Albert Roy Davis, Ph.D., noted that positive and negative magnetic polarities have different effects upon the biological systems of both animals and humans. Davis then concluded that negative magnetic fields have a beneficial effect on living organisms, whereas positive magnetic fields have a stressful effect. A positive magnetic pole, with prolonged exposure, interferes with metabolic functioning, produces acidity, reduces cellular oxygen supply, and encourages replication of latent micro-organisms. Positive magnetic fields can increase pain due to their interference with normal metabolic functions.

Robert Becker, M.D., found that weak electric currents promote the healing of broken bones. He brought national attention to the fact that electromagnetic interference from power lines and home appliances can pose serious hazards to human health.

Kyoichi Nakagawa, M.D., Director of the Isuzu hospital in Tokyo, Japan, believes that the time people spend in buildings and cars reduces their exposure to natural geomagnetic fields of the earth, and may interfere with their health. He calls the condition that they subsequently must suffer from, magnetic field deficiency syndrome, which, he says, can cause headaches, dizziness, muscle stiffness, chest pain, insomnia, constipation and general fatigue.

According to William H. Philpott, M.D., of Choctwaw, Oklahoma, magnetic fields can stimulate metabolism and increase the amount of oxygen available to the cells of the body. Dr. Philpott pioneered the use of magnetic therapy for psychiatric disorders. The biological value of oxygen is increased by the influence of a negative electromagnetic field, and the field causes the negatively charge deoxyribonucleic acid (DNA) to "pull" the oxygen out of the bloodstream and into the cell. The negative electromagnetic field keeps a cellular buffer system (pH or acid-base balance) intact so that cells remain alkaline; pathogenic microorganisms cannot survive in a well-oxygenated, alkaline environment. Also, magneto therapy can increase enzyme action because it fosters a favorable environment within cells (mainly a proper pH).

An electromagnetic field (EMF) is composed of both an electric and a magnetic field. The electric field is due to the presence of charged particles (such as electrons) and the magnetic field is due to the movement of the charged particles (such as an electron current).

Static magnetic fields are produced by natural or artificial magnets. Pulsating magnets are generated entirely by electrical devices.

Magnetic Resonance Imaging

Magnetic Resonance Imaging (MRI) is slowly replacing x-ray diagnosis because it is safer and more accurate. The most significant use of magnetic energy in conventional medicine is through MRI. A sophisticated diagnostic tool, MRI employs the different effects of the two Poles on the hydrogen factor in human tissue to create an image otherwise unavailable. The MRI system detects and details soft tissue and is important in detailing the brain and detecting tumors. Teeth and bones that contain little water do not appear on an MRI image. Other approved devices include EEG, MEG and SQUID diagnostic equipment, which can also detect and record important electromagnetic information. In addition, magnetoencephalo graphy is now replacing electroencephalography (EEG) as a preferred technique for recording the brain's electrical activity.

Other Applications

Other applications using magnetic and electromagnetic energy are infrared heat therapy equipment, ultraviolet purification systems, magnetic hearing aids, and homoeopathic, colour and light therapies. Kinesiology test equipment and magnetic probes which remove metal particles from the eyes, nose and ears can also be included.

While some diseases and disorders respond best to orthodox medicine, conventional medicine and alternative therapies can work in harmony. Natural alternatives are generally safer with fewer side effects and should be considered whenever possible.

Benefits of Biomagnets

As we enter the 21st century, the most promising pain relief therapy is biomagnet therapy. Compared to these other pain relief therapies, biomagnet therapy has at least six advantages causing its explosive, worldwide growth today.

1. Biomagnets relieve the root cause of pain, not just the symptoms only.
2. Biomagnets are safe. They have no known side effects since our bodies already live in the earth's natural, magnetic field.

3. Biomagnets are simple. Anyone can use them in the privacy of their own home.
4. Biomagnets are non-consumable. You don't have to buy another bottle or schedule another appointment every month!
5. Biomagnets work quickly, often in only a few minutes, sometimes in weeks.
6. Biomagnets are affordable. Especially since you can use them, again and again, for years.

And this is only the beginning. The history of magnet therapy is a fascinating account of a famous queen, philosophers, doctors and scientists. For thousands of years magnet therapy has been advancing toward its latest discovery of the newest and most powerful biomagnets.

Use of Magnetometer

There are no harmful side effects to magnetic field therapy if used properly. A magnetometer is used as a standard method of determining the poles of a magnet. With a compass, the arrowhead of the needle marked "N" or "North" points to the magnets negative pole. The strength of a magnet is measured in units of gauss (magnetic flux intensity) or tesla (1 tesla=10,000 gauss). The actual strength of a magnet at the skin surface is less than the manufacturer's gauss rating because the magnet's strength decreases with increasing distance from the subject.

Two different conventions or "standards" for naming the north and south poles of a magnet have developed. One is called the "conventional" or "industrial" magnetic pole nomenclature, while the other is called the "magneto biological", "biomagnetic", or "medical" convention. Unfortunately, they are opposite to each other: What the industrial convention calls north, the medical convention calls south and vice versa.

Use of Magnetic Products

Large machines capable of generating high magnetic fields are used for treating fractures and pseudoarthritis, a joint affliction caused by nerve breakdown. Magnetic blankets and beds reduce stress and promote sleep. Ceramic, plastiform and neodymium (rare earth chemical element) magnets are placed individually or in clusters above various portions of the head.

In Japan, small tai-ki magnets are designed to stimulate acupuncture points, although no clinical studies have been done on these magnets as of yet. Small disc magnets (made or ceramic neodymium or iron oxide) are placed around the head to alleviate symptoms of panic, seizures, delusions and hallucinations.

Methods of Magnetic Therapy Application

There are generally two different methods of magnetic therapy application, those who expose the body to only the north (negative) pole and those who use low gauss strength simultaneous exposure to both the negative and positive poles. Magneto therapy practitioners who exclusively use the north (negative) pole suggest an exposure intensity of 2,000 to 4,000 gauss, an intensity not recommended for a dual or bi-polarity applications.

The placement is generally simple and straightforward, with the magnet being placed directly on the area being treated, like applying a band-aide. In contrast, magneto therapy practitioners who promote the use of spatially alternating magnetic poles generally employ magnets that are made with some sort of spatial pattern of alternating magnetic polarity such as concentric circles or a checkerboard pattern.

Magneto therapy uses electromagnets and permanent magnets.

Magnetic field is produced in electromagnets only when electric current is passed through them. When the current flow is stopped, magnetic field disappears. On the other hand, permanent magnets remain magnetized permanently even after the electric current is disconnected.

Mostly disc shaped magnets are used for treatment. These discs are sold in pairs, i.e. north pole and south pole. The two poles possess different healing properties.

The north pole is helpful in curing diseases caused by bacterial infection. On the other hand, the south pole is used to treat all kinds of pains, stiffness and weakness.

For the treatment, both the poles are placed under the palms or soles. The north pole is applied to right side and south pole to the left.

Duration of Treatment

The duration of treatment is very important.

Generally, a magneto therapy session lasts for about half an hour. Even after the ailment is cured, the treatment can continue. Magnetised water is also strongly recommended as it acts as a tonic.

In serious ailments, the longer a magnet is applied to the injured or painful area, the more quickly it heals and the greater the symptom relief. Close to twenty-four hours a day application is sometimes suggested, if possible. The duration of treatment is dependent upon the persistence of symptoms.

Benefits of Magneto Therapy

1. Many health problems, once diagnosed by the medical profession, can be treated effectively and safely by the patient using magnets without resorting to potentially dangerous drugs.
2. The use of magnets is simple and the benefits can be immense. Magnets aren't magic. Their use isn't quackery.

3. Magnets have been scientifically proven to be able to assist the body regain its self-healing electromagnetic balance naturally.
4. Magneto therapy is basically helpful in relieving pain and stiffness from the body. When the human body comes in contact with magnets, the magnetic waves pass through the tissues. As a result, currents are induced which lead to the production of heat thereby reducing pain.
5. We all are aware that hemoglobin in our blood contains iron. By attracting iron, the magnetic effect reaches the whole body. This helps in removing harmful minerals and cholesterol from our body.
6. A negative magnetic field applied to the top of the head has a calming, sleep-inducing effect on brain and body functions, due to the stimulation of the production of the hormone melatonin. Melatonin is antistressful, antiaging, antiinfectious, anticancerous, and has control over respiration and the production of free radicals (highly destructive molecules that are missing one electron, and readily react with other molecules). Free radicals can lead to decreased efficiency of protein synthesis.
7. Dr. Albert Roy Davis found that magnets could be used to arrest and kill cancer cells in animals, and could be used to treat arthritis, glaucoma, infertility, and diseases related to aging.
8. Magnets eliminate toothaches, eliminate periodontal disease, and eradicate fungal infections, like candidiasis.
9. Magnets dissolve kidney stones and calcium deposits in inflamed tissues.
10. Furthermore, magnetic therapy reduces swelling and oedema.

11. A negative magnetic field can stop such symptoms as hallucinations, delusions, seizures or panic without disrupting a patient's mental alertness.
12. The negative magnetic field normalises disturbed metabolic functions that cause painful conditions such as cellular acidosis (excessive acidity of cells), lack of oxygen to cells, and infection.
13. Magnets possess the power to purify blood. They ionize blood due to which it flows easily without any obstructions. This in turn helps in proper functioning of the cardiovascular system.
14. If there is any hormonal imbalance, then magnets can go a long way in treating the same.
15. And if or body has a balanced secretion of hormones define, the skin glows with radiance.

The common cures are:

1. Osteoporosis
2. Fractures
3. Joint disease
4. Rheumatoid arthritis
5. Temporomandibular joint syndrome (TMJ)
6. Muscle tension
7. Hypertension
8. Circulatory diseases
9. Heart disease
10. Diabetes
11. Epileptic seizures
12. Optic nerve atrophy
13. Parkinson's disease (There are motor and non-motor benefits of magneto therapy)
14. Headaches and migraines
15. Insomnia and sleep disorders

16. Environmental stress
17. Multiple sclerosis
18. Migraine and other headaches
19. Environmental stress
20. Breast cancer
21. Post-surgical swelling
22. Cranio-facial pain
23. Pain after operations
24. Inflammations

Popularity of Magneto Therapy

Magnetic devices are very popular in Germany because the use of certain devices is covered there by medical insurance. NASA eventually incorporated artificial magnetic fields inside manned spacecraft because of the realisation that the earth's natural geomagnetic fields are probably beneficial and perhaps necessary to life itself.

With MRI and other magnetic field diagnostic techniques, magnets and electrical devices are beginning to gain mainstream medical acceptance as human diagnostic and treatment tools because medical equipment manufacturers and distributors are primarily driven by the profit motive to promote their products. Because magnets do not introduce any foreign substances to the body, this will make them safer over the long-term than aspirin or other over-the-counter medications.

The repeatedly observed benefits of magnetic field therapy, while intriguing, are too often not convincing to many Western medicine authorities and practitioners. In order to rule out placebo effects and convince mainstream doctors that magnetic field therapy actually does work, many scientific studies need to be done and published in reputable, peer reviewed journals. This means that placebo studies with both real and fake (placebo) magnets must be done.

As of now, there has been little funding for magnetic field therapy, an important area of science and medicine.

The best part is that magneto therapy is not habitual and does not produce any side-effects.

Magneto therapy can work wonders for your health. But along with that regular exercise and a balanced diet is a must.

❖❖❖

14
Massage Therapy

Wide Use of Massage Therapy

Massage Therapy is a rapidly growing field of treatment for relief of stress and other ailments due to muscle tension or strain. In the fast-paced world that we live in, unfortunately, stress is a part of most of our everyday lives.

The purpose of massage therapy is to prevent, develop, maintain, rehabilitate or augment physical function or relieve pain.

Massage therapy is recogniaed as one of the oldest methods of healing, with references in medical texts nearly 4,000 years old. It is a widely accepted and effective treatment for reducing stress, decreasing muscle pain and stiffness, and for aiding in rehabilitation and postural realignment.

Benefits of Massage Therapy

Massage therapy can be tremendously beneficial for people of all ages and conditions. While it is known best to benefit the ill, the injured and the stressed, massage is also a great treatment in preventing illness and conditions before they develop.

Massage therapy not only treats those parts of you that are a problem, but also affects your whole body. It is not only your muscles that are treated during a massage, but also your circulatory and nervous systems. This helps to restore an overall feeling of well being.

Many of today's health problems arise from stress. Because stress upsets the delicate balance of all your body's functions, regaining this balance requires a holistic (whole body) approach.

Stress is a very troublesome presence in our lives. In severe, prolonged situations stress may even cause death. Regular massage therapy treatment will reduce the effects of stress on our lives and be a welcomed relief that enables us to live more fulfilling lives. Not only is massage therapy helpful in relieving the ailments caused by stress, but also symptoms which accompany certain syndromes and diseases. If you are unsure if massage is right for you please check with your family physician before receiving massage therapy.

Adults and children alike can benefit from massage therapy. Infants can be relieved from symptoms of colic, gas, constipation and discomforts. Parents may want to attend infant massage therapy classes to learn infant massage. Infant massage is also quite effective for the premature baby. Bonding and attachment, and relaxation are also benefits that the parents and infant will receive from infant massage.

There are tremendous benefits to be achieved through regular massage therapy treatments from a registered massage therapist. Whether your need is to have a moment of relaxation, reduce muscle tension or attain relief from chronic pain, a therapeutic massage can enhance your overall sense of emotional and physical well-being as well as your quality of life.

Massage therapy benefits people of all ages. While it benefits the injured, the ill and the stressed, the strength of massage therapy in preventing illness and conditions before they develop cannot be overlooked. Massage therapy can be used in the treatment of both acute and chronic stages of conditions.

During treatment, the physical therapist may include localised massage (e.g. low back or neck) as a prelude to exercise. Massage increases circulation and warms muscles and other soft tissues (e.g. tendons, ligaments).

Other types of massage include full-body massage, which often leaves the patient feeling relaxed and free of anxiety.

Guidelines to Follow Before and After a Massage Therapy

Before massage you may want to empty your bladder as massage rids the body of toxins which are present. After the massage you will need to drink plenty of water to flush out these toxins. Toxins enter our muscles through different ways. Some medications which we take for pain or symptom relief leave behind residue which deposits into our muscles causing muscle tightness or sometimes spasms. Also, muscle dehydration caused from lack of sufficient water intake can cause the muscles to tighten and spasm, so be sure to drink plenty of water (6 to 8 glasses a day is recommended).

As the therapist uses his/her hands or specialised tools to rhythmically knead, rub and stroke (effluerage) muscles, circulation is stimulated. Blood flow delivers oxygen and nutrients, and is key to helping muscles eliminate waste products such as lactic acid that may collect in muscles from spasms causing pain.

Following trauma, muscles may act as mini-splints to protect and limit motion, similar to a cast on a broken arm. A typical example is a person who uses a computer for a prolonged time period without taking a break to stretch the neck. The result: stiff neck, aching, even pain. Taking periodic breaks to rub (mini-massage) and stretch the neck will promote circulation to the muscles.

Types of Massages

There are various types of massages that are beneficial to everyone.

Swedish Massage

The Swedish Massage is the most popular form of massage used in most countries. Often a lotion or oil is used to reduce skin friction. The therapist combines light stroking in one direction with deep pressure in another to relax muscles. The treatment expedites blood flow to flush lactic acid, uric acid and other waste products from the muscles. Ligaments and tendons are stretched increasing their suppleness, nerves are stimulated and relaxed, and stress is alleviated. The overall goal is to relax muscles.

Deep Tissue Massage

The Deep Tissue Massage technique targets chronic muscle tension. The therapist's strokes are slower using more direct pressure and friction. Depending on the texture of the deeper layers of muscle and tissue felt, the therapist periodically adjusts his/her hand positions, strokes and intensity to work the tissues to release tension.

Myofascial Release

Myofascial Release, or soft tissue mobilisation, is a therapy used to release tension stored in the fascia. Fascia are sheets of fibrous tissue that encase and support muscles separating them into groups and layers. Following trauma, the fascia and muscles may shorten restricting blood flow. The techniques used in myofascial release relax muscle tension and break up fascial adhesions.

Trigger Point and Myotherapy

Then there is the Trigger Point and Myotherapy. Trigger points are tiny tight nodules that form in muscles causing referred pain. Sometimes myofascial pain can be linked to one or more trigger points. The treatment goals include alleviating muscle spasms, improving circulation, and releasing trigger points. The therapist applies direct momentary pressure to a trigger point to cause its release. During the massage, the therapist may return several times to a stubborn trigger point to elicit its release.

As trigger points are released, the therapist stretches the muscle using a technique called Spray and Stretch. This technique incorporates a superficial cooling agent such as fluori-methane, a local anesthetic that depresses nerve response. The anesthetic is sprayed over muscles as they are gently stretched soothing tight muscles.

Shiatsu, Reiki and Rolfing

There are many, a few are mentioned here. Shiatsu is an old oriental therapy based on acupressure, as is Jin Shin Jyutsu.

Reiki is a Japanese form of massage that seeks to adjust the body's energy.

Rolfing can be uncomfortable; the goal is to adjust the muscle fascia to its fullest extension.

Facelift Massage

The Facelift Massage is a specialised massage therapy treatment which actually improves the muscle tissue and promotes conditioned facial muscles to reduce sagging skin and improve muscle tone. The facelift massage system offers a solution to anti-aging. When you receive a facelift massage session your facial muscles are toned and tightened and the skin softened and you will enter into a state of deep relaxation..... Sheer Bliss!

Pregnancy Massage

Pregnancy Massage is a welcomed relief from the stresses of pregnancy on the body and muscles. The client lies on her left side with pillows around her, which is quite comfortable; massage is applied to the back, arms, legs, feet or any specific problem area for the expectant mother. It is very relaxing, while increasing circulation and reducing oedema. Check with your doctor before receiving pregnancy massage.

Lymph Drainage Therapy

Lymph Drainage Therapy (LDT) is an original hands-on method of lymphatic drainage developed by Bruno Chikly, MD, of France. LDT is very gentle. It is not painful — the touch is very light. Specially trained therapists work with flat hands, using all the fingers to simulate gentle, specific, wave-like movements. These subtle manual maneuvers activate lymph and interstitial fluid circulation as well as stimulate the functioning of the immune and parasympathetic nervous systems. Lymph is fluid that circulates just beneath the surface of the skin. The main functions of the Lymphatic System are to absorb excess fluid to cleanse tissue on a regular basis and remove waste and cells in acute conditions such as an injury or necrosis. Through this process the lymphatic system maintains optimal functioning and retains the integrity of the connective tissue and regulates the fluid volume and pressure in a tissue.

Trigger Point Massage

The Neuromuscular Therapy or Trigger Point Massage is a deep tissue massage focusing on points of spasm in muscles causing deep pain that may also refer to other areas of the body. Especially effective for headaches and jaw pain. Injuries that have long healed can still cause muscle spasms. This therapy may help alleviate the pain. Trigger points from everyday use of the body's musculature can be deactivated.

Sports Massage

The Sports Massage is excellent for sports enthusiasts and athletes. Pre-event massage can assist in improving performance. Post-event massage aids in recovery of the muscles.

Swedish Skin Exfoliation

The Swedish Skin Exfoliation, a refreshing and invigorating massage uses soft abrasive gloves and body shampoo to knead tired muscles and remove old skin cells. The session leaves your skin smooth and glowing, and your body and mind fresh and alert.

Lypossage

Lypossage, an extremely precise combination of deep tissue and lymphatic drainage modalities, enhances firmness and tone, increases skin resilience and smoothness, and reduces the appearance of cellulite. it reduces dimension and improves muscle tone producing a lifting effect in many areas prone to sagging, including the buttocks, upper arms and lower face. Lypossage can be used in combination with body wraps or without.

Hot Stone Massage Therapy

In the Hot Stone Massage Therapy, the use of heated stones is combined with traditional massage techniques to create a beneficial and relaxing experience. Heated stones are placed on your body to relax muscles while other stones glide along tired and sore muscles. Hot stone massage has many benefits including increased circulation, and the flushing of toxins from the body and facilitating more effective deep tissue work.

Corporate Chair Massage

For the Corporate Chair Massage the therapist will come to your worksite with a specially designed chair to give a 10 to 15 minute massage on employees' necks, arms, backs, and hands. This provides a refreshing break and productivity booster.

Benefits of Massage Therapy

The following is a list of conditions for which massage therapy can prove beneficial:

1. Anxiety and depression
2. Asthma and emphysema
3. Back, neck and shoulder tension
4. Breast tenderness/inflammation
5. Cancer
6. Carpal tunnel syndrome
7. Cerebral Palsy
8. Chronic Fatigue syndrome
9. Circulatory problems
10. Digestive/lower bowel problems
11. Dislocations

12. Fibromyalgia
13. Fractures
14. Frozen shoulder
15. Gastrointestinal disorders
16. Headache/ Migraine
17. Inflammatory conditions such as arthritis and bursitis
18. Insomnia
19. Kyphosis and scoliosis
20. Low back pain
21. Multiple sclerosis
22. Muscle spasm
23. Neuritis/neuralgia (nerve pain)
24. Oedema (inflammation)
25. Parkinsonï's disease
26. Muscle tension and spasm
27. Palliative care
28. Post-injury rehabilitation
29. Post-surgical rehabilitation
30. Pregnancy and labour support
31. Respiratory problems
32. Repetitive train Injuries
33. Sciatica
34. Sports injuries
35. Strains and sprains
36. Stress and stress related conditions
37. Stroke
38. Tendonitis
39. Whiplash

Therapeutic massage is an important part of your health maintenance plan. It assists in:

1. Reducing or eliminating pain
2. Improving joint mobility
3. Improving circulation
4. Improving immune system functioning
5. Increasing lymphatic drainage
6. Reducing depression and anxiety
7. Reducing tension within muscles

Massage therapy benefits people of all ages. While it benefits the injured, the ill and the stressed, the real strength of massage therapy lies in prevention.

If you have any of the following conditions please consult your family physician before receiving massage therapy:

1. Osteoporosis
2. Varicose Veins
3. Phlebitis
4. Aneurosa
5. Hematoma
6. Oedema
7. High Blood Pressure
8. Cancer
9. Chronic Fatigue
10. Heart or Lung Disease
11. Diabetes
12. Asthma

There are some situations where massage therapy is absolutely not appropriate, such as in severe cases of uncontrolled hypertension, shock, acute pneumonia, acute stages of rheumatoid arthritis, or toxemia during pregnancy.

A massage should be a relaxing, pleasurable experience. The pain or pressure felt during some types of massage should always be temporary. Finding the right therapist and the appropriate style can be daunting. Massage Therapy offers a drug-free, non-invasive and humanistic approach based on the body's natural ability to heal itself.

❖❖❖

15
Mud Therapy

What is Mud Therapy?

Mud therapy is a venerated health tradition based on the warm, external application of volcanic or hot springs clay mud to treat certain diseases and injuries, and to promote health and well being.

Mud is one of five elements of nature having immense impact on the body in health as well as in sickness. It can be employed conveniently as a therapeutic agent in naturopathy treatment as its black colour absorbs all the colours of the sun and conveys them to the body.

Mud therapy is a new version of beauty treatment. Many people are not familiar with the mud therapy. But in short we can say that mud therapy is recent mode of beauty enhancement. It also helps to cure many ailments.

The mud is a mixture of an organic solid component mixed with mineral water which is then left for several months to "mature".

The mud is heated to 50°C and then applied to the body. The client is then wrapped up to stop any heat dispersion. The client finishes the treatment with a therapeutic thermal bath or shower followed by 10-15 minutes of relaxation.

It originated with ancient societies located near volcanoes, lakes and the ocean that, after intuitively using mud as a means of body camouflage to blend in with the environment, gradually become aware of its therapeutic properties. They observed how this special mud soothed muscular aches, alliviated joint stiffness and pain - later understood to be associated with arthritis and rheumatism - and improved skin conditions. In time, they realised that the earth was offering them a priceless gift.

Mud contains a much higher concentration of minerals than hot springs waters since it is formed by the long-term accumulation of the residues from these waters, which rise to the surface carrying both dissolved and undissolved compounds from deep inside the earth.

Mud therapy is the safest of all therapies of all other kind of holistic therapies as it does not have any side effects. Various spas all over the country carry out the mud therapy treatment.

Mud is one of the five elements of nature having immense impact on the body in health as well as in sickness. It is used as the best therapeutic agent in naturopathy treatment. Various methods and treatments have been defined in the *Vedas* for the ailing. Mud was and is supposed to be one of the most beneficial remedies of all times.

The difference between mud therapy and thermal baths is the concentration of minerals, since in the former it tends to be larger and, in general, those of a volcanic origin present a larger proportion in sulfur.

Varieties of Mud Used for Therapy

Mud consists of 53 per cent clay, 36 per cent minerals, 4 per cent water and 7 per cent organic materials and is said to reduce aches and pains, relieve swollen joints, and even prevent these ailments.

There are four varieties of mud being used for health and rejuvenation purposes: moor mud (the most common), volcanic mud, mud from thermal springs, and mud extract from the base of the ocean.

Mud procured for treatment purpose should be black cotton soil with greasiness and free from pollution and contamination.

Before use mud should be dried, powdered and sieved to separate stones, grass particles and other impurities.

Earth to be used for treatment must be obtained from ant- hills or river beds. It must be pounded well and sieved to remove stones or coarse particles of sand in it.

The naturopathy practitioners use moistened earth to cure diseases.

Usually mud therapy is done in two ways - Mud Packs and Mud Bath.

Mud Pack

Mud is supposed to be a rejuvenator of the body and when it is mixed with sandal, it comes out as one of the best beauty secrets. Mud is best used for the skin therapies. The mud pack is supposed to calm down the senses and rejuvenate the body and mind. It also acts as secret for youthful skin with no wrinkles. The mud retains the moisture of the body intact, open the pores of the skin to let it breathe, relives internal congestion and pain and promotes elimination of morbid matter,

The mud pack is prepared by the clay obtained from about 10 cms below the surface of earth, after ensuring that it does not contain any composite or any pebbles. The clay is then mixed with water and a paste is made out of it. This when cooled down is spread on a cloth which is then applied as per requirement of the treatment.

Mud packs have been found to be a valuable treatment of diseases relating to general weakness or nervous disorders.

Mud pack is prescribed for swellings, eye troubles, gout, rheumatism, stomach troubles, kidney disorders, headache, etc.

Mud pack is also useful as an alternate treatment. The area under treatment is first given fomentation for five minutes until it is well heated. Mud is then applied directly to the skin for fifteen minutes, depending on the reaction required.

When applied to abdomen it relieves all forms of indigestion. It is effective in decreasing intestinal heat and stimulates peristalsis. A thick mud pack applied to head in congestive headache relieves the pain immediately. The advantage of mud pack cold over compress is, retains the coolness for a longer time. Hence, this is recommended whenever there is necessity for a prolonged cold application.

Mud Bath

Mud or clay bath is another mode of treatment. It is applied in the same way as packs, but only on a larger scale on the entire body. A cleansing water bath and a cold shower follow a mud bath.

It is given in a special cubicle where the patient can expose himself to sunlight. Mud may be applied to the patient in a sitting or lying position. A massage is done and when the clay gets dried up its washed off with cleansing water bath. This helps to improve the skin condition by increasing the circulation and energiaing the skin tissues. Care should be taken to avoid catching of cold the bath. Afterwards, the patient must be thoroughly washed with cold water jet spray. If the patient feels chill, warm water is used. The patient is then dried quickly and transferred to a warm bed

The mud bath is useful for toning up the skin by improving the blood circulation. The mud bath is especially useful in getting temporary relief from rheumatic pain or pains caused by injuries or accidents. Usually the duration of the bath is from 20 to 30 minutes.

Hot and Cold Mud Therapy

The Mud Therapy also makes use of the Hot and Cold Mud Therapy. This Therapy is helpful in reliving chronic pains, intestinal cramps and lumbago. Others like amoebiasis, colitis, enteritis and other inflammatory conditions of bacterial origin are also treated by the Hot and Cold Mud Therapy.

Hot and cold applications are useful in relieving chronic pains, intestinal cramps and lumbago. Alternate application helps to relieve discomfort caused by flatulence and intestinal obstructions. It is also helpful in colitis, enteritis and other inflammatory conditions of bacterial origin.

Benefits of Mud Therapy

1. Mud therapy involves the use of mud in packs or baths to treat and also prevent pathologies in the joints and fortify the organism to combat stress.
2. Mud reduces inflammation and improves circulation, absorption, and elimination. When it is applied on an affected part it soothes the inflammation and painful part.
3. The mud is used to help treat osteoarthritis, rheumatism, periarthritis, back and joint aches and pains where there is no inflammation.
4. It is also a great purifier as it draws away toxins from the system by increasing circulation in the affected part where it is applied.
5. Mud therapy is also useful to lose weight, detoxify, and tonify and revitalise the skin.
6. Mud therapy is normally carried out once a year and lasts an average of one to two weeks. When using a mud pack, the mud is soaked in a thin, wet muslin cloth and made into a thin flat brick. The pack is applied for about 20 to 30 minutes. When applied to the abdomen, the pack relieves indigestion. When applied to the head, it relieves pain from headaches.
7. For complexion problems, a soaked mud paste is applied on the face and allowed to dry for 30 minutes. This is

helpful in removing pimples and eliminating dark circles around the eyes.

8. Mud also helps in clearing the dark spots on the face, is good for patients suffering from heat or heart burn and helps in treating diseases like psoriasis, leucoderma and even leprosy.
9. In mud baths mud may be applied to the patient in sitting or lying position to help circulation as well as to improve the skin condition. The scrubbing effect exfoliates the surface of the skin leaving it smooth and rejuvenated.
10. Mud therapy is used as an exclusive technique in rheumatic diseases and in skin ailments (psoriasis, acne, etc.) and in esthetics, taking care of the kind of skin they are applied on, since mud with a high mineralisation in sulphur dries and reddens sensitive skins.
11. Mud baths are also recommended for skin diseases such as psoriasis, urticaria, and other allergic conditions. We know of the good results got for dermatological ailments, an example of these are some studies developed by dermatologists. The cold moisture in the mud relaxes the pores of skin, draws blood to the surface. It restores proper skin pH'
12. Mud can be used for rheumatic pathologies: arthritis, rheumatism, etc. because it produces surface heat diminishing the muscle spasm, joint inflexibility and a possible anti-inflammation action.
13. According to some studies, mud restores magnesium and other minerals for the formation of substances which are important in the development of muscles and diminishing muscular pain.
14. Besides, mud produces the activation of some enzymes, as well as the incorporation of substances called oligoelements which are necessary for some metabolic functions: zinc, cobalt, copper, manganese, etc., are some of them.

15. As the mud retains moisture for a long time, when applied over the body part it causes cooling.
16. It relieves internal congestion and pain.
17. It helps in acne repair and prevention.
18. No drugs are involved and so there are no side effects.
19. It aids in natural hormone balancing due to peat.
20. Its shape and consistency can be changed easily by adding water. Moreover, it is cheap and easily available.
21. Mud therapy retains moisture for longer time than cold-water pack.
22. Mud therapy is anti-inflammatory and anti-aging.

In short, mud therapy is used therapeutically for:

1. ***Joint problems:*** To reduce inflammation and absorb edemas
2. ***Muscular problems:*** To supply magnesium and phosphorous, boosting the energy level of the muscles so that lactic acid is eliminated, thus alleviating aches and pains
3. ***Skin conditions:*** To treat such problems as psoriasis and acne, and to prevent premature aging; nourishing the skin cells with minerals can help to increase their enzymatic activity, revitalising tissues

Mud contains magnesium and phosphorous, which have a tensing effect on the skin - ideal for restoring elasticity and for treating cellulite - and silicates, which help to leave the skin baby smoothIn general, the treatments with mud can be developed with masks or face applications, occlusive or subocclusively, depending on the patient's skill and the ailment to be treated.

Mud therapy, as shown by experience, has no big incompatibilities, except it must not be used in open wounds, no hot mud in serious processes, so it is recommended medical supervision before mud therapy or thermal baths.

Application of Masks

The application of masks, generally, is recommended twice a week or depending on the ailment to be treated, in those cases of occlusive application. For chronic rheumatic pathologies they can be used once a day and in general with temperatures that go from 35ºC and 38ºC, getting a local vessel dilation that favours mineral absorption.

Who Should Avoid This Therapy

It is actually harmless. But people having following problems should avoid mud therapy:

1. People having sensitive skin should avoid it because sensitive skin may get upset due to mineral water used which is rich in sulfur.
2. People suffering from claustrophobia may get irritation on the cuts and sores
3. Pregnant ladies should use only after the consulting her doctor that her unborn baby will not have any risk

Side Effects

Because the temperature of the mud can reach about 100 degrees Fahrenheit, water will be drained from the body and can cause dehydration. If you have sensitive skin, the warm mud may cause skin irritation. It is important to be monitored by a spa professional while taking a mud bath because staying in the bath too long can cause heat stroke, nausea and fainting.

Prevention/Solution

In order to prevent negative side effects from occurring, drink plenty of water the day before and several hours before having mud bath therapy. If you have never had mud bath therapy before and you have sensitive skin, ask to have a portion of the mud painted on the inside of your arm in order to determine if you will have a reaction.

Identification

While in the mud bath, if you are feeling dizzy, light-headed, itchy, overheated or uncomfortable, contact someone to help you get out of the mud bath. If you are alone, slowly push yourself out of the mud bath, standing up slowly. If you are seeing stars or feel like you are going to pass out, attempt to roll out of the mud bath and onto the floor where you can call for help.

Warning

Frequent mud bath therapy can cause severe dehydration. Unless recommended by a doctor, it is not necessary to have a mud bath more than once a week. Mud baths can be draining on your system so it is important to drink plenty of water before and after having mud bath therapy.

❖❖❖

16

Ozone Therapy

What is Ozone Therapy?

Everyone needs to become aware of alternative therapies regarding their health and to choose which they feel is best to fight disease. Without free choice we have nothing,

The combination of oxygenation and oxidation is ozone therapy. Ozone therapy is a therapy which is used as one of the hottest new age healing systems. It is not a new technology. These applications have been in use around the world by alternative health care professionals and in veterinary clinics for over fifty years. It has been proven to work by doctors and veterinary clinics for bacteria and viral infections, and pain with the lowest side effects in existence,

When the human immune system is at its peak with proper oxygen levels it can prevent many disease and other health problems. Ozone therapy can revitalise the practice of medicine with alternative therapies that work because of its antibacterial, anti-fungal, anti-inflammatory, anti-parasitic, anti-tumour and antiviral.

Ozone and oxygen therapy is one of the most powerful and versatile therapies known today. Research shows it throughout the twentieth century, mostly in Europe and other parts of the world. The action of ozone has beneficial effects on every part and organ. Some of the effects are bacterial, fungal and viral inactivation, circulatory enhancement, disruption of tumor metabolism, and stimulation of oxygen metabolism.

Using ozone therapy, it is extremely important that you receive all the positive effects and not become dissatisfied from its use. It will work for you, if you apply it properly. The success of this depends on retaining the mixture of gas and allowing it to absorb through the colon.

Role of Oxygen in Therapy

Oxygen plays the most vital role for an optimum immune system and maintaining health. Oxygen, along with food, is the primary nutrient that cells use to generate energy for all its functions. With oxygen, the energy production is through oxidation of the unhealthy cells.

Oxygen regulates all activities of our bodies. Our ability to think, feel, and act comes from the energy created by the oxygen. Approximately 90 per cent of our energy originates from oxygen. The oxygen we breathe in is our most vital element for good health.

Benefits of Ozone Therapy

1. Ozone therapy is harmless when used properly and has virtually no side effects. It is one of the most effective ways of restoring optimal levels of oxygen. Its actions have beneficial effects on every part that will stimulate the bodies immune system.
2. Ozone therapy has many applications within the medical and veterinary clinics where bacterial and viral cross contamination are problems that need to be addressed in many doctors offices and hospitals throughout the world. The spread of fungal or yeast infection, parasites, tuberculosis and other airborne infectious disease can be minimised when using an ozone generator.
3. Oxygen therapies have many therapeutic uses that have beneficial effects on every part of our bodies. Ozone

therapy is recognised by most as the most powerful versatile therapy known in alternative health because it plays vital roles in maintaining our well-being.

4. Oxygen along with food is the primary nutrient that cells use to generate energy for all its functions. This energy is produced through oxidation of the unhealthy cells.

5. One of the most important aspects to note about the ozone therapy is the breadth of its therapeutic usefulness. It is useful and valuable for so many different symptoms and health issues. For instance we can use its antioxidant stimulating capabilities, its anti-viral, anti-bacterial and anti-fungal properties.

6. Ozone is also an immune system modulator, and has powerful analgesic properties.

7. From a naturopathic perspective, ozone supports body detoxification, and helps with cleansing the lymph system.

The other benefits are:

1. Ozone removes unwanted bacteria and viruses from the blood, the same way it does with water.

2. The possibility of becoming infected with hepatitis, HIV virus, syphilis or other infectious diseases through blood transfusion could be eliminated by the use of ozone.

3. Ozone is highly effective in peripheral vascular disease.

4. Ozone is effective in cardiovascular and cerebro-vascular disease, arteriosclerosis and hypercho-lesterolemia, and promptly restores circulation, relieves angina pain and improves brain function.

5. With ozone cancerous tumors, lymphomas and leukemia may be eliminated without the use of surgery, radiation or chemotherapy.

6. Ozone is highly effective for all forms of rheumatoid and arthritis collagen diseases.
7. Ozone is very effective for allergies of all types.
8. Ozone improves multiple sclerosis, and other neurological diseases, senility, as well as in Parkinson's disease.
9. External use of ozone is very effective in treating burns, acne, leg ulcers, open cuts and wounds, eczema, fungus and other skin disorders.
10. Rectal insufflation with ozone is effective for proctitis, colitis, prostatitis and fissure; vaginal insufflation is effective for candidiasis and other yeast infections, trichomoniasis and other forms of vaginitis; bladder insufflation is effective for cystitis and bladder fistulas, as well as cancer.
11. AIDS, herpes, hepatitis, mononucleosis, and cirrhosis of the liver have been successfully treated with ozone.
12. The application of ozone is virtually painless. It has no adverse side effects and is extremely cost-effective for both physicians and patients.
13. Ozonated water helps when you are suffering from viral infections such as cold, flu and virus.

Ozone Generators

The use of ozone generators is well documented for most all health conditions and various ailments and others like parasites, staphylococcus and fungal infection. Oxidative therapy is routinely practiced in countries such as Germany and Switzerland. Since the legality of ozone generator's and their applications vary from country to country, check with your physician and your local legal authority before embarking on any alternative. Legality is not an issue in veterinary clinics for pets.

Range and Methods of Ozone Therapies

There are a range of simple and safe methods of ozone therapy.

The simplest and most enjoyable ozone therapy is an ozone sauna. This involves sitting and relaxing in a steam cabinet (just surrounding your body and limbs - not your head), while ozone is pumped into the unit at the correct therapeutic amount.

As you relax, all your body, (except your neck and head) will be bathed in an ozone oxygen steam mixture. The steam moistens and warms your skin, opening your pores and allowing the ozone to gently penetrate and oxygenate your tissues.

The ozone oxygen steam mixture will also act as an anti-bacterial, anti-yeast and anti-viral agent on your skin surface.

As well as the benefits of the ozone, this method is advantageous in that raising the body temperature slightly is beneficial in terms of stimulating the immune system and helping the body detoxify.

Also one extra benefit may also be that you lose a little weight because during a 25-30 minute session in the cabinet, your body will use up approximately 500 calories.

Sometimes other methods of ozone therapy are indicated, for instance, cupping. Briefly, cupping is an ozone therapy which involves concentrating ozone over over a particular area of the body. For instance, an infected wound, or an organ that is diseased, such as breasts, prostate or liver, may benefit from cupping over the area.

It is usually best to start with the ozone sauna, and move on to the other forms of therapy later if they are appropriate, but, obviously as an individual you have your own needs and requirements.

Another method of inhalation in low concentration is through room air purifiers. This method is the simplest for absorbing it into the lungs and circulatory system.

If you are suffering from spinal injuries like low back pain and disc disorders, you can use injections of ozone gas, ozonucleolysis or ozone discectomy which will provide you better results than surgery.

Ozonucleolysis treatment is less painful and cost effective. Ozone discectomy is the injection of ozone and this is injected into affected intervertebral disc.

Method for absorbing ozone through the skin is by injecting it into an ozone resistant suit below the neck. Plastic bag can be used for the arm, leg or foot and sealing it off tight with the tube inside.

Most will stay inside the suit for 30 minutes. Before getting in the bag or suit, it is best to take warm or hot shower and remain damp. This opens the pores and allows the gas to absorb at faster rates.

Some people use it in the ear for one minute each, three times per day, or three minutes in each ear, alternating every minute. This method is called auricular insufflations.

Some people with arthritis problems will fill plastic buckets or smaller containers with warm water, large enough for the foot or hand and let the activated oxygen bubble under the limb for about five minutes. The warm water opens the pores allowing it to penetrate. After the first or second application, itching may occur. You should experience movement without stiffness or pain soon after with minor arthritis problems.

Other topical applications have been used on bruises, burns, fistula, decubitus, gangrene, infections, muscle pains, radiation damage, and used to promote the healing of wounds.

Some prefer the 25-day program of oral treatments using 35 per cent food grade hydrogen peroxide for cleansing. They usually start with 3 drops mixed in an 8-ounce glass of non chlorinated pure water, juice or milk and taken 3 times per day. Dosage is increased by 1 drop per day as they work up to 25 drops 3 times per day.

Its essential to provide your bodies with the necessary supplements during any oxygen therapy. OXY-MEGA colon cleanser and liquid vitamin and mineral supplements will accelerate the efficiency of ozone therapy and stimulate the internal cleansing and healing process.

Slight heating sensation is felt as the activated oxygen is oxidizing the germs. Heat may be more noticeable in the vagina and the ear. The heating sensation is only temporary.

Some may experience minor rashes or itch on the skin as the system is dumping out the toxins and going through the cleansing effect. Some will increase with their oxidative therapies for faster elimination of the accumulated debris.

When you increase your detoxification, you also need to increase your vitamin-mineral (especially electrolytes) supplements and vitamin E. Eating fresh vegetables and drinking lots of water will help flush out the waste from the intestines at faster rates.

Benefits of Ozonated Water

Ozone is the only natural alternative to purify water. Research shows drinking ozonated water helps allergies, cold sores, headaches, gastritis, gum disease, mouth ulcers, thrush, ulcers, yeast infections, increases circulation, reduces infections after dental work, helps remove free radicals, helps colds, flu and virus, cleans wounds and minor bruises. It also helps in reducing infections after dental work. Drinking ozonated water also increases the oxygen level throughout and accelerates the healing process.

Ozone is also used as natural alternative for purifying water. If you drink the ozonated water, it will help you when you are suffering from allergies, carcinoma, cold sores, headaches, gastritis, gum disease, mouth ulcers and yeast infections.

Ozonated water also helps in increasing circulation. It also helps in cleaning wounds and minor bruises.

Ozonated water helps in increasing oxygen level in your body and for accelerating the healing process.

Benefits of Hydrogen Peroxide

Hydrogen peroxide (H_0O_2) is one natural by-product of most ozone oxidizing processes. Hydrogen peroxide is another great natural alternative for your health.

There are three methods used for administering hydrogen peroxide to detoxify; orally, intravenous and through colonic irrigation. These applications are called Oxidative Therapies. Diseases that have benefited from this oxidative therapy are heart and cardiovascular, pulmonary, infectious and immune diseases; in addition, Parkinson and Alzheimer.

Some physicians are injecting ozone directly into cancer tumors or into the muscle (Intra-muscular) for treating infections. Injecting it into the blood through the portal vein (Intra-arterial) may cause some adverse effects in some people.

Benefits of Autohemotherapy

Another method, which purifies the blood of bacteria and infectious disease causing mycoplasmas, is called autohemotherapy. About 50 to 100 ml is withdrawn and mixed with medical ozone and then reintroduced by intravenous drip back into the patient. Autohemotherapy will cause the inflammation of vein, circulatory depression, chest pain, shortness of breath, fainting, cardiac arrhythmia and gas embolus (bubble in the blood will lodge and block the blood beyond the bubble). Autohemotherapy (ozonation of blood) will help in treating AIDS, arthritis, hepatitis, allergy and herpes.

Benefits of Ozonated Products

1. Lemon, orange and aloe vera juice can be ozonated for drinking or applications to the skin. By ozonating two cups of fresh lemon juice for six hours (use larger container because of the bubbles) has been used on all skin conditions like dry skin, psoriasis and ulcers.
2. Ozonated olive oil has many therapeutic uses and benefits. Its used as topical applications for dry skin and beauty aid for wrinkles, and for treatment of sunburn. It can be inhaled directly when bubbled through the olive oil. Ozonated olive oil works when applied for cuts, bruises and other conditions.
3. Using ozonated steam in cabinets is currently being used around the world for alternative health by aesthetician, chiropractors, massage therapists, and other practitioners because they recognise this natural way to detoxify and cleanse. Ozonated steam stimulates circulation and increases the oxygen supply.

How does Ozone Work?

1. Inactivation of bacteria, viruses, fungi, yeast and protozoa

Ozone disrupts the integrity of the bacterial cell envelope through oxidation of the phospholipids and lipoproteins. In fungi, ozone inhibits cell growth at certain stages. With viruses, the ozone damages the viral capsid and disrupts the reproductive cycle by disrupting the virus-to-cell contact with peroxidation. The weak enzyme coatings on cells which make them vulnerable to invasion by viruses make them susceptible to oxidation and elimination from the body, which then replaces them with healthy cells.

2. **Enhancement of circulation**

   In circulatory disease, a clumping of red blood cells hinders blood flow through the small capillaries and decreases oxygen absorption due to reduced surface area. Ozone reduces or eliminates clumping and red cell flexibility is restored, along with oxygen carrying ability. Oxygenation of the tissues increases as the arterial partial pressure increases and viscosity decreases. Ozone also oxidises the plaque in arteries, allowing the removal of the breakdown products, unclogging the blood vessels.

3. **Stimulation of oxygen metabolism**

   Ozone causes an increase in the red blood cell glycolysis rate. This leads to the stimulation of 2,3-diphosphoglycerate (2,3-DPG) which leads to an increase in the amount of oxygen released to the tissues. There is a stimulation of the production of the enzymes which act as free radical scavengers and cell wall protectors: glutathione peroxidase, catalase, and superoxide dismutase. Ozone activates the Krebs cycle by enhancing oxidative carboxylation of pyruvate, stimulating production of ATP. Ozone also causes a significant reduction in NADH and helps to oxidise cytochrome C. Prostacyclin, a vasodilator, is also induced by ozone.

4. **Formation of peroxides**

   Ozone reacts with the unsaturated fatty acids of the lipid layer in cellular membranes, forming hydro peroxides. There is a synergistic effect with cellular- formed H2O2. Lipid peroxidation products include alkoxyl and peroxyl radicals, singlet oxygen, ozonides, carbonides, carbonyls, alkanes and alkenes.

5. **Dissolution of malignant tumours**

Ozone inhibits tumour metabolism. In addition, ozone oxidises the outer lipid layer of malignant cells and destroys them through cell lysis (break-down). Phagocytes produce H2O2 and hydroxyl to kill bacteria and viruses. The generation of hydroxyl by killer cells is critical to their cytotoxic capability. Ozone stimulates conversion of L-arginine to citrulline, nitrite and nitrate by phagocytes, acting on tumours.

❖❖❖

17
Reflexology

What is Reflexology?

Reflexology, or zone therapy, is the practice of stimulating points on the feet, hands or ears, in the belief it will have a beneficial effect on some other parts of the body, or will improve general health. Most scientists and medical professionals consider reflexology to be a pseudoscience, offering no more benefits than ordinary massage.

Reflexology is based on a system of zones and reflex areas that reflect an image of the body on the feet and hands with a premise that such work effects a physical change to the body.

History of Reflexology

Around the world and throughout history reflexology has been rediscovered and reinstated as a health practice time and time again by peoples around the globe seeking to deal with health concerns. Archeological evidence Egypt, China and Japan points to ancient reflexology medical systems.

Eunice Ingham developed Reflexology in the 1930s, based on earlier theory by Dr. William Fitzgerald known as "Zone Therapy". In 1913, Dr. Fitzgerald noted that specific parts of the body could have an anesthetic effect on another area. Developing this theory, he divided the body into ten equal vertical zones, ending in the fingers and toes. He concluded that pressure on one part of the zone could affect everything else within that zone.

In the West the concept of reflexology began to emerge in the 19th century, based on research into the nervous system and reflex. While no direct evidence of direct cross-fertilisation from ancient times has been discovered, the practice of foot and hand work in a variety of cultures, belief systems and historical periods speaks to reflexology for health as a universal bridging concept.

Foot Reflexology

Reflexology is a widespread practice in Asia, where foot reflexology (also known as foot massage) is quite popular. Although many people are sceptical about the concepts underlying this practice, its use is spreading, perhaps because it is being taken simply as a relaxing massage therapy. It is not the practice that reflexologists use foot reflexology only, they prefer to use a combination of foot, hand and ear reflexology to obtain a much better result.

It could be argued that all bodywork is reflexive, therefore reflexology. We find that the extremities have a powerful influence because of locomotion. While we acknowledge that repeated patterns exist throughout the body we find our most effective focus to be the feet and hands.

Pressure is applied to the feet and hands using specific thumb, finger and hand techniques. Stretch and movement techniques are utilized as "desserts" to provide relaxation to the foot.

The most common form is foot reflexology. Practitioners believe the foot to be divided into a number of reflex zones corresponding to all parts of the body, and that applying pressure to tight or "gritty" areas of a person's foot will stimulate the corresponding body part and cause it to begin healing itself.

The body is reflected on the feet or hands. Left foot/hand reflects the left side of the body and the right foot/hand the right side.

The spine reflex area runs down the insides of the foot and hand with reflex areas for the arm and shoulder reflected toward the outside of the foot or hand.

The toes and fingers reflect head and neck reflex areas as well as those of the internal parts of the body they enclose.

The ball of the foot mirrors the chest and upper back in addition the heart and lungs.

At the base of the long bones of the feet and hands is represented the waistline of the body.

Portions of the body above its waistline are mirrored above this line toward the toes or fingers and those below the waistline toward the heels of the foot or hand.

Internal organs lying above the body's waistline are reflected by reflex areas above this line while those below the waistline are mirrored below this line.

Reflexologists apply pressure on "reflex zones" found on the feet, hands and the ears, which are said to correspond to the different parts of the body. Application is done through thumb, finger and hand technique. Reflex areas, like hand and foot, composed of 7,200 nerve endings are stimulated by pressure applied. An improved instruction to every gland, single part and organ of the body could be achieved by such a health science. The body is then believed to pursue a biologically correct, strengthened and reinforced state. The reflex zones are organised in a way that represents the whole body.

Role of the Vital Energy

In reflexology, it is believed that there is a "vital energy" that is circulating between organs of the human body, that penetrates into every living cell. Whenever this energy is blocked, the zone of blockage will be affected, and the reflex zones can indicate the blockage of energy in different organs. Therefore, if someone has a problem in a particular organ, a reflexologist will press on the corresponding reflex zone or zones, and the person will experience pain.

This pain is claimed to originate from the deposition of crystals in the reflex zone and, with massage, these crystalline structures can be broken down and the pain relieved. Simultaneously, the pressure applied to the reflex zones by the reflexologist is claimed to pass through the nerves to dissipate energy blocks.

Benefits of Reflexology

For the most of the part, the sensation is pleasant and soothing. Reflexology can help relax the client and is believed to stimulate the body's own healing mechanisms. Usually a treatment session lasts for about one hour. For some cases, a treatment can last nearly two hours. A course of treatment varies in length depending on the need of the client body.

In general terms the benefits of reflexology have to do with the reduction of stress. Because the feet and hands help set the tension level for the rest of the body they are an easy way to interrupt the stress signal and reset homeostasis, the body's equilibrium.

Whether reflexology can benefit certain conditions and diseases is still under investigation. Further scientific study need to be done in order to come to some definite benefits of reflexology in regard to illness and disease.

Reflexology assessment takes place as stress cues are evaluated. Stress cues are parts of the foot or hand that shows adaptation to stress. Adaptation is shown by visual signs such as callousing, knobby toes or bunion. Indications of stress are also seen as sensitivity to technique application or touch signs perceived by the reflexologist as technique is applied. The assessment of such stress cues allows the reflexologist to target areas of stress and to design a session of pressure technique application appropriate to provide relaxation specific to the individual.

Reflexology can be done practically anytime and anywhere. The trick is consistency. We have been impressed with the results from China. Their secret seems to be that they do reflexology once a day for six days in two week segments. Then they review the results and do more segments as necessary.

This requires self-help and family help as well as the guidance of practitioners. The practitioner can give you a quality signal to break up the pattern of stress but you and your family can provide the quantity to help break it up the stress patterns in your feet and hands.

Foot Reflexology Equipment

Sales of foot reflexology equipment, such as rollers, are increasing rapidly. In addition, many new instruments using the same principle are being marketed, such as whole body vacuum cans. Socks printed with reflex zone footmaps were developed based on reflexology. By wearing the socks, people can easily locate appropriate areas to apply pressure to. Though not generally used by professionals, these "reflexology socks" have gained popularity in Taiwan and China.

Inexpensive how-to books enabling people to perform the exercises by themselves are also available for self-help practice. Reflexologists advise caution in applying the techniques to oneself, and recommend people to consult an expert before using them if they are pregnant or have a chronic disease.

Advocates claim reflexology is just as effective when used on children as on adults. Some advocates go further and claim it is more effective. Advocates have also suggested that reflexology can also help children create an awareness of self.

Criticisms Regarding Use of Reflexology

Most scientists and medical professionals consider reflexology to be a pseudoscience and claim there are no reliable scientific studies proving its effectiveness as a medical treatment, or that there is any form of link between specific areas of the feet and the various organs of the body.

Furthermore, the 'crystalline structures' rationale is unsustained by current understanding of physiology. There is no scientific evidence that healing can be achieved by it or that the claimed "energies" and their supposed pathways through the body even exist. However, research shows the relaxing and pleasurable nature of massage has many medical benefits.

Prominent sceptic Stephen Barrett, M.D., contends there is no scientific support for any of the theories of reflexology, and refers to several scientific studies that have shown reflexology is no better than random chance detecting medical problems. In a paper titled "Reflexology: A Closer Look", Dr. Barrett concludes: "Reflexology is based on an absurd theory... Claims that reflexology is effective for diagnosing or treating disease should be ignored. Such claims could lead to delay of necessary medical care...."

William T. Jarvis, Ph.D. says: "Reflexology has almost no potential for direct harm, but its ability to mislead well-meaning people into believing that it can be used for screening for health problems, or that it has real therapeutic value could lead to serious problems.

Reflexology is a complement to standard medical care. It should not be construed as medical advice. It should not be a replacement to medical help. So please use it wisely.

Build reflexology into your life. It is easy to do reflexology well doing other activities. Put a foot roller under your desk or work your hands while waiting for the kids at school. Be creative but be consistent. Five minutes a day is worth more than an hour once in awhile.

18
Water Therapy

What is Water Therapy?

Water therapy is a natural treatment for controlling diseases and keeping the body hydrated. Since diseases first began to plague the earth, man has continuously looked for the perfect medicine to cure all the sickness. At the same time, man is also looking for a way to prevent all the possible sickness for people to live longer and experience life to the fullest.

These ambitions of man have led to the development of medicine as we know it. Surgeons have become more specialised and expert in very sensitive areas of the human body such as the heart and the brain. These people can now operate without any fuss on a brain of a human or even the live pumping heart of man in the operating room. At the same time, there are also alternative medicines being developed and introduced to the public such as herbal capsules and herbal therapies.

There is one alternate therapy being introduced to the public and being constantly supported by various practitioners. This therapy is practically free, safe and can be done without the help of any specialist. The therapy is called Water Therapy.

Water therapy supports free and safe treatment. The water therapy treatment is done without the help of any specialist. This water therapy is used when you require perfect medicine to cure all sickness.

Water is Life

Water is a precious gift to mankind and forms almost 70 per cent of our body weight. Therefore can you imagine how important water is for the smooth functioning of the body systems.

Water therapy is the natural alternate treatment that can be followed by any person at any age of your life time. Water without life is impossible and you can live longer with water. The treatment with water is very simple and you can follow this therapy at your own place.

When you reach home tired from work the only thing you want first is water. Nothing else refreshes better than a glass of cool water. Water is a very essential part of our life. It is a major constituent of our body and even of the earth. You may have been told by many people and doctors that drinking lots of water is very essential for your body. Water regulates different functions of body. It helps in digestion of food and formation of new blood. Life is incomplete without water.

Have you ever wondered how can water add quality to our life? Water possesses disease curing properties. By using water therapy many dreadful diseases like breast cancer, kidney stone, asthma etc. can be prevented. Along with allopathy and homoeopathy the new option of water therapy is also available. Water therapy has proved that 'water is life' indeed.

Water also keeps the digestive tract in order and helps to flush out the toxins and controls constipation.

No wonder then that water acts as a natural remedy towards achieving a beautiful and healthy skin.

We get water in abundance and yet fail to grasp the worth of it. Plenty of water in your daily day diet will show glowing health results. To stay healthy, drink water in plenty. Water flushes sodium from our body and it kills the bloat.

Do's and Don't's of Water Therapy

Water therapy is helpful in curing diseases without using medicine. Water Therapy is really simple. If you wish to undergo water therapy, prepare 1.5 litres of water everyday. Then drink them altogether and fast for at least an hour from any food or drink and that's it. You may wonder why 1.5 litres. It's the estimated amount of water you can take so that you body can be cleansed with the use of water. Everyday the water will clean all the toxins found in your body and release them via sweat or urinal excretions. It is a natural remedy for most diseases.

You can prevent and even get rid of health problems by only drinking water. All you have to do is strictly follow these instructions:

1. Drink 1.5 litres or 5-6 glasses of water as soon as you get up in the morning. You can wash your face and brush your teeth after drinking water.
2. Start with drinking 3-4 glasses of water if you are unable to drink 5-6 glasses of water in the beginning.
3. Avoid taking alcoholic beverages the previous night.
4. Avoid eating or having any other drink one hour before and after drinking water in morning.
5. Drink water thrice a day if you are suffering from arthritis or rheumatism. You should drink 1.5 litres of water each time. You should continue this routine for one week. After one week you can drink 1.5 litre twice a day till the disease is cured.
6. Consult your doctor to find out whether water therapy will suit your body or not if you are ill or are already having a health problem.

Water therapy is so simple that it does not require expert supervision or professional guidance. Have a quick look at benefits that can be gained with the help of water therapy. It will almost feel like water is a magical drink.

Lack of sufficient water causes:

1. Dehydration
2. Difficulty in blood circulation
3. Body gets less active and more tired.
4. Dehydration due to decreased water intake or increased loss by way of evaporation leads to premature ageing. In this, the dehydrated skin shows in the form of fine lines and dryness.
5. Constipation due to low water intake as we all know leads to raised toxin levels and therefore a dull skin that easily breaks out into pimples.
6. The right amount of water is necessary for skin's elasticity and suppleness. Even without sweating the body is losing water through the skin and this needs to be replaced. Otherwise the skin cells become dry, crack, peel and change colour.

Water has the power to hydrate, revitalise, detoxify and oxygenate the skin. Increased warm water intake regulates the excess oil present in an 'acne- prone' skin.

Water for Skin Care

Let us just enumerate some of the basic needs of water in skin care.

The hygiene in our body especially skin starts with a soap and water bath. Hygiene prevents body odour, fungal infections and any other parasitic or bacterial infection.

Detoxification and weight regulating programmes use a lot of water in their treatment protocols. Large amounts of water need to be consumed in both these treatments. This in turn flushes away toxins, clears constipation, increases immunity of the body and thus affects the skin directly.

Then come the skin care products that use water as their base. These products (sunscreen, moisturisers, body lotions, repair serum, night creams) are used to prevent or reverse the cutaneous ageing of the skin.

Many exercises also use water, e.g., swimming, floatation therapy, steam hydrotherapy, etc, that increase blood flow to the skin and which in turn increases levels of nutrients and oxygen and flushing off of toxins that again imparts a glow to the skin. Healthy cooking also requires water.

Thus we can easily say that 'water is life' and the secret of a glowing skin is "water, water everywhere and lots of it to drink".

Dangers of Water Therapy

Before we look into its effects, let's all consider first the danger of this therapy. People have shown hesitation to this kind of therapy since there is a potential of water intoxication – a fatal disease that can happen from drinking water. This can be prevented by drinking clean waters and give intervals in drinking the whole 1.5 litres.

People also showed hesitation since drinking 1.5 litres will make you urinate from time to time. This is true, however, with daily intake of water; the body would eventually adjust to the water intake and you can act normally even with the daily intake of 1.5 litres every day.

Benefits of Water Therapy

Now let's take a look at the benefits water therapy has to offer.

1. If taken properly, constipation can go away with only one session.
2. Acidity is known to be cured with only two sessions.
3. Diabetes can be controlled with only seven sessions.
4. Hypertension can be controlled with only four weeks of water therapy, and even cancers are known to be controlled in the same amount of time.
5. If person has pulmonary TB, three months of water therapy should do it. These facts were based on research and experience by followers.

6. It suppresses appetite.
7. It metabolises fat into energy.
8. Water helps muscle stimulation.
9. Lots of water will reduce body fat deposition.
10. Kidneys function properly with good water intake.
11. Water pampers the liver too.
12. It helps dehydration and relaxes us.
13. Water dissolves nutrients such as oxygen and minerals to the body.
14. It flushes the toxins from the body.
15. Burning calories is a process which requires water in good quantities.
16. Water therapy helps to control anemia, rheumatism, general paralysis, obesity, arthritis, sinusitis, tachycardia, giddiness, cough, leukemia, bronchitis, meningitis, hyper acidity, dysentery, gastroenteritis, uterus cancer, rectal piodapse, eye-disease, ophthalmic halmorrhage, irregular menstruation, laryngitis, headache and many other diseases.

The properties of water are helpful in some of the following conditions:

1. The physical properties of water are used for treating back pain and other musculoskeletal injuries.
2. Buoyancy of water will help the patient to support weight and will improve your balance and strength.
3. The viscosity of water provides resistance by its gentle friction. It will help in strengthening and conditioning of an injury and reduces the risk of injury due to loss of balance.
4. Hydrostatic pressure of water has powerful effects to improve heart and lung function. This pressure is useful for maintaining and strengthening heart and lung

function. This pressure will effect in improving muscle blood flow.

5. Water is a zero-calorie drink. So substitute it with fruit juices or soft drinks and take the first step towards a weight loss goal. If you drink enough water regularly you can lose up to two kilos a week. Increase your weight loss by taking cold water as your body needs to heat up the water generating calorie loss. Drink water when you are hungry between meals or just before one. Even if you are fit and not aiming for a weight loss, don't lose touch with water therapy as it is good for each one of us. Also, it's free of cost, easily available, natural, with no side effects and good for health.

Always Consult Your Physician

This is actually an amazing therapy. However, if you are seriously ill, make sure to contact your physician first and get their confirmation before chugging down this volume of water. Sometimes there are patients who are advised against drinking too much water as they would be harmful to their own health. But if you're not a special patient and see no complications in your body, start drinking and see the results in no time. You'll feel healthier, stronger and cleaner inside and out.

Water Therapy Exercises

There are various water therapy exercises that are found to be beneficial to us. Water therapy exercise programmes (sometimes called pool therapy, hydrotherapy, or aquatic therapy) consist of a variety of aquatic-based treatments and exercises that are designed for back pain relief, to condition and strengthen muscles.

Water therapy exercise offers many of the same benefits associated with a land-based exercise programme, including development of a treatment plan that is carefully tailored to the individual.

Water therapy exercise is especially helpful in cases where a land-based exercise programme is not possible due to pain, decreased bone density, disability or other factors. As such, water therapy is a versatile exercise and is particularly good for people with conditions such as:

1. Osteoarthritis
2. Advanced osteoporosis (with susceptibility to and/or pain from fracture)
3. Muscle strain or tears

In addition to those conditions, water therapy is frequently recommended as one form of exercise therapy to treat those with diabetes as well as individuals with high blood pressure. Both conditions can improve and become more manageable with aquatic exercise. All of these conditions can make it uncomfortable or painful to exercise on a hard or even padded surface, or while standing. Water provides a much gentler, welcoming environment.

Benefits of Physical Properties of Water

The physical properties of water make it a highly desirable medium in which to exercise to treat back pain and other musculoskeletal injuries. Some of the most important properties of water that make exercise easier are:

1. ***Buoyancy:*** water counteracts gravity and helps to support the weight of the patient in a controlled fashion as the patient is immersed. This can aid the development of improved balance and strength.
2. ***Viscosity:*** water provides resistance by means of gentle friction, allowing strengthening and conditioning of an injury, while reducing the risk of further injury due to loss of balance.
3. ***Hydrostatic pressure:*** there are powerful effects produced by hydrostatic pressure that improve heart and lung function, making aquatic exercise a very useful way to maintain and strengthen heart and lung function. This pressure effect also aids in improving muscle blood flow.

Together, these properties allow development of an exercise regimen that minimises the weight placed on the spine (axial load) and risk of injury due to unintended movements during exercises. For example, individuals with osteoarthritis in the neck (cervical spine) and shoulder could practice arm circles or shoulder rolls in water to improve their range of motion and strength. Because the water provides both mild resistance and support through buoyancy, the person would most likely not experience the pain caused when a tired arm drops suddenly, as it can do at the end of land-based exercises.

Moreover, the perception of pain may be diminished as a result of many factors including the relaxing sounds as well as the warmth of the water during water therapy exercise, making it a different and often very pleasurable experience.

Finally, the buoyancy of water permits a greater range of positions due to the virtual elimination of gravitational forces, particularly for exercises that require lifting the legs, the heaviest limb of the body for most people.

Exercises such as range of motion stretches for hip flexors and abductors are generally much easier to try out first in water because the leg is supported somewhat as the individual learns the right positioning. Buoyancy when doing water therapy exercises can be increased with the use of floats.

Active techniques for water therapy back exercise are diverse and should be tailored to the individual. Exercises range from simple routines performed in a shallow pool to conditioning using underwater treadmills and other high-tech equipment.

Water therapy exercises muscles and joints, as well as the back.

Water therapy for back exercise can be a short-term exercise option if back pain or a back injury makes land-based exercise too difficult. Or it can be adopted as part of an ongoing exercise program if land-based methods worsen symptoms or if the person prefers water exercises. If their functional status or competitive goals require it, people may transition to exercise in a dry environment once they are successfully performing exercises in water.

Some people may find mixed use of wet and dry exercise therapy environments most beneficial.

There is a small but growing body of scientific studies demonstrating the benefits of aquatic exercise in the management of spine pain. Although more scientific evidence for the specific benefits of water therapy exercise in treating back pain will be helpful in creating specific programs for particular spine problems, the value of appropriate aquatic exercise programs is well established overall and has been beneficial in many thousands of individuals. The aquatic medium is ideal for patients for whom land-based options for back exercise are limited, and may provide a safe and effective method of managing spine pain while improving function.

Who should not use Water Therapy

For many back pain patients, water-based exercises should only be performed under the guidance of a qualified health professional. Water therapy exercise should usually be avoided if a person has any of the following:

1. Fever
2. Severe heart failure
3. Incontinence
4. Infection

Individuals with severely limited endurance or range of motion may not be able to safely navigate a tiled (and slippery) pool apron to participate in a water therapy exercise program. Rubber mats are often used to increase traction to reduce this risk.

The perception of objects (like the instructor demonstrating exercises) in water is also affected by refraction, leading to difficulty in learning specific motor skills in patients with limited eyesight, or impaired sense of body position or balance due to stroke or other injury. Also, the water temperature may be too warm to accommodate some conditions.

Therapy is generally conducted in pools or tanks with water that is between 90 to 94 degrees (Fahrenheit), almost as warm as bath water, so blood circulation is increased. Consequently, patients with any of the conditions listed above should avoid or limit their water therapy exercise, or make sure the pool or tank used is cooler so that their conditions are not exacerbated.

Finally, for patients with low bone density or osteoporosis, the buoyancy provided by the water may not be as beneficial for building bone as weight bearing land-based exercises although the added strength and balance achieved through an aquatic exercise programme may facilitate a safe return to land-based exercise.

Spa Therapy and Treatments

The techniques used in water therapy exercise for back pain include spa therapy, standing or floating pool exercises, swimming, and conditioning using specialised equipment, such as surgical tubing, flotation devices and resistive devices for the hands or feet.

Spa treatments complementing water therapy back exercise typically involve relaxing in warm, agitated water such as that found in whirlpool baths. This form of hydrotherapy relaxes muscles, improved muscle blood flow and increases general blood circulation, which make the body more flexible and can prepare it for water therapy or land-based exercise.

Pool Therapy Exercises

Some of the basic techniques for pool therapy exercises are as follows (they can be modified for varying degrees of difficulty:

1. ***Knee-to-chest exercise.*** This movement is performed with one hand on the side of the pool or with back to the wall. Alternating between legs stretches the lower back, as well as the gluteus (buttocks), quadriceps (front thigh) and hamstring (back thigh) muscles.

2. ***Leg raise exercise.*** This movement is performed with one leg outstretched and the supporting leg slightly bent while one hand holds onto the side of the pool. It strengthens and stretches the muscles in the leg, hip and lower back.
3. ***Wall-facing leg stretch exercise.*** In this stretching exercise individuals assume a "Superman" position with hands resting on side of pool and the body and legs outstretched into and supported by water. This extends all regions of and joints in the back as well as stretching shoulder muscles.
4. ***Pool walking exercise.*** Walking both forward and backward in chest-high water works the leg muscles while exerting no impact of the knees or hips, particularly important for people who have arthritis in those joints. The walking exercise can be made more demanding with the addition of hand floats or light weights, so a stroll in the pool becomes an aquatic version of power walking.
5. ***Quadruped activity and exercise.*** This exercise works legs and arms and is performed while floating on one's back (sometimes achieved with a therapist supporting the trunk or using a flotation jacket). The individual makes paddling motions with his/her arms and legs.

Precautions

When you do not have a limit for doing things they may become a threat. Too much of a good thing can also pose a harm. This is true in the case of water therapy also. When water intake is not controlled while undergoing water therapy it may cause danger. It is because our body has limited capacity of throwing the excessive water. If this limit is crossed, body can face critical condition known as water poisoning or hyper hydration. This can expose a human body to the risk of brain damage or heart failure.

So to avoid any risk you should always consult professional or doctors before undergoing any such therapy. It is important to know the pros and cons of any treatment, diet or therapy that you plan to take up. Practise water therapy according to given instructions and avoid overdoing it. Remember, too much of anything can be bad. Maintain a balance and enjoy the goodness of the wonder drink called, water.

❖❖❖

19

Traditional Chinese Medicine

What is Traditional Chinese Medicine?

Tongue and pulse diagnosis, Chinese herbs, nutrition, and acupuncture comprise the ancient practices of Traditional Chinese Medicine (TCM).

With a history of 2000 to 3000 years, Traditional Chinese Medicine (TCM) has formed a unique system to diagnose and cure illness. The TCM approach is fundamentally different from that of Western medicine. In TCM, the understanding of the human body is based on the holistic understanding of the universe as described in Daoism, and the treatment of illness is based primarily on the diagnosis and differentiation of syndromes.

TCM has even more recently become a respected alternative therapy worldwide during the last decade. Unknown to many, Traditional Oriental Medicine is a major healthcare system for over one quarter of the world's population. Cited as an effective system of healthcare by the National Institute of Health and the World Health Organization, acupuncture and Oriental Medicine are becoming a serious alternative or complement to conventional pain management and medical treatment.

Oriental medicine is an effective, low cost medical treatment that works in harmony with the body's natural healing ability. Diagnosis in Oriental medicine involves the classical procedures of observation, listening, questioning and palpation, including feeling pulse quality. Treatment focuses on the well-being of the entire person, not simply on the physical complaints and symptoms.

A TCM diagnosis is holistic in nature. The practitioner trained in Traditional Chinese Medicine will take into consideration all the aspects of the individual, including special observation of the tongue and the wrist pulses. These two areas (among others), according to TCM, tell the practitioner about certain characteristics of the person regarding their overall constitution. These findings tell the practitioner what treatment is needed.

Consequences of Imbalance in Vital Energy

According to the theories of traditional Oriental medicine, all the disorders or diseases from which people suffer can be related to an imbalance in one's *Qi*, or vital energy. Oriental medicine's aim is to improve the patient's health both physically and spiritually by rebalancing the body's own healing mechanisms.

The TCM approach treats zang—fu organs as the core of the human body. Tissue and organs are connected through a network of channels and blood vessels inside human body. *Qi* (or *Chi*) acts as some kind of carrier of information that is expressed externally through jingluo system.

Pathologically, a dysfunction of the zang-fu organs may be reflected on the body surface through the network, and meanwhile, diseases of body surface tissues may also affect their related zang or fu organs.

Affected zang or fu organs may also influence each other through internal connections. Traditional Chinese medicine treatment starts with the analysis of the entire system, then focuses on the correction of pathological changes through readjusting the functions of the zang-fu organs.

The Chinese culture, philosophy, and even their language makes explanations of "vital energy" or "Qi" within the body plausible, and for the most part, unquestioned. For the Chinese, "*Qi*" is no more mysterious than electricity. Anything that helps "move" this vital energy when it is stagnant will help bring the body back into balance or homeostatis, thus allowing it to heal.

Syndromes

Evaluation of a syndrome not only includes the cause, mechanism, location, and nature of the disease, but also the confrontation between the pathogenic factor and body resistance. Treatment is not based only on the symptoms, but differentiation of syndromes. Therefore, those with an identical disease may be treated in different ways, and on the other hand, different diseases may result in the same syndrome and are treated in similar ways.

Various TCM Therapies

The typical TCM therapies include acupuncture, herbal medicine, and qigong exercises. With acupuncture, treatment is accomplished by stimulating certain areas of the external body. Herbal medicine acts on *zang-fu* organs internally, while qigong tries to restore the orderly information flow inside the network through the regulation of *Qi*.

These therapies appear very different in approach yet they all share the same underlying sets of assumptions and insights in the nature of the human body and its place in the universe. Some scientists describe the treatment of diseases through herbal medication, acupuncture, and qigong as an "information therapy".

The Yin-Yang Theory

The clinical diagnosis and treatment in Traditional Chinese Medicine are mainly based on the yin-yang and five elements theories. These theories apply the phenomena and laws of nature to the study of the physiological activities and pathological changes of the human body and its interrelationships.

The principle of Yin /Yang in Chinese philosophy is simple, but to understand such a "foreign" concept, Westerners have written numerous books on the subject. Originally, the "Yang" was the sunny side of a slope, and the "Yin" was the shady side of the slope. These terms are used to describe any item in nature. When the two forces are in balance, the item being described is in its natural state. It Yang is described as "hot", the Yin must be described as "cold"; if Yang is "outside", then Yin is "inside"; if Yang is "up", then Yin is "down"; if Yang is the "head" of a coin, Yin is the "tail" of the coin, etc.

In the exercise system of Taijiquan, the practitioners upset this balance in their opponent while maintaining their own Yin/Yang balance. Whenever one of the forces increases to its extreme, a violent transition will occur to bring them back into balance (this is where the legends of extraordinary strength originates).

It is important to realise that Yin and Yang are not separate items, they always appear together when speaking about the principles of Yin/Yang. Since one is opposite, yet complimentary of the other, one cannot appear without the other. In fact, the presence of one without equal amounts of the other is exactly what Acupuncture and Acupressure is designed to correct. When there is a condition in the body where the Yang force is excessive, then an acupoint that either reduces the Yang of this force, or an acupoint that increases the Yin of this force is stimulated.

Either of these treatments will balance the two forces of Yin and Yang, thus bringing the body back into its natural "balance" or state of homeostatis. When the body is in a state of homeostatis, it is considered healthy. The selection of what acupoints to use and whether to increase or decrease forces in the body is difficult and why acupuncturists go through rigorous training, and have access to thousands of case studies.

Five-Element Theory

There are several schools of theory within the modern Acupuncture community. One of the most popular is the theory of the Five Elements. Proponents of this system use the relationship of five elements and the meridians or channels of energy in the human body to bring forces back into balance. For instance, if their diagnosis shows an excessive Yang condition in an energy related to a "fire" element, they may look for the cause as being either a Yin or weak condition in the "water" element (not enough water to control the fire), or they may find an Yang condition in the "wood" element (too much wood feeding the fire).

Now when you consider the "fire" as the heart, the "water" as the kidneys, and the "wood" as the liver, you can begin to see how a typical treatment may be configured. This also explains the reason why the Acupuncturist may ask a lot more questions than a typical Western physician as they inquire about seemingly unrelated topics. A Western physician would seldom ask if you have trouble urinating or other kidney-related questions like a craving for salt when you go for a heart checkup, yet surprisingly, Western science has led to many similar conclusions (excessive salt can be bad for your heart).

The theory itself is simple but the relationships and diagnosis can become quite complex with creation cycles and destruction or controlling cycles, etc. Most body functions are divided into Yin/Yang tendencies, then subdivided into elements or qualities.

Another important difference in Eastern and Western medicine is that every traditional Oriental diagnosis is individual and unique. Two persons with the same symptoms may receive completely different treatments because the cause of their "imbalances" may be different. Oriental medicine looks for the "causes" of the disease, not necessarily treating the symptoms directly.

Acupuncture

Acupuncture (Zhen Jiu) and Acupressure (Zhi Ya) are the most well-known of all traditional Chinese methods of healthcare worldwide, especially in the West.

It is important to understand that Acupuncture (and Traditional Chinese Medicine in general), is not "folk medicine". It is a highly developed, systematic, recorded, researched, and peer reviewed form of medicine with several disciplines that continues to evolve. It has a massive amount of real-world data to justify the application of techniques based on several thousand years of human trials.

Throughout the world, lay-persons have adopted the techniques far more readily that scientists because they do not have to understand how it works to take advantage of it. From janitors to high-profile quarterbacks, the word is out-it's cheap, it's painless, and most importantly-it works.

Over 2000 acupuncture points on the human body connect with 14 pathways, called meridians. Chinese medicine practitioners believe these meridians conduct energy, or *Qi*, between the surface of the body and internal organs. *Qi* regulates spiritual, emotional, mental, and physical balance. When *Qi* flow is disrupted, through poor health habits or other circumstances, pain and/or disease can result. Acupuncture acts to keep the normal flow of this energy unblocked.

Acupuncture is the insertion of hair-thin, disposable metal needles through the skin in points on the body's meridians. Acupuncture needles are solid, usually made of stainless steel and extremely flexible. Inserted a few millimeters into the skin, the small diameter and contoured shape of the acupuncture needle allows it to be inserted easily and painlessly. Acupuncture needles can also be stimulated with pressure, heat, friction or electromagnetic impulses to further activate a person's *Qi*. Acupuncture involves the insertion of fine needles through the skin and tissue at specific points on the body. There is no injection of any substances, and the treatment itself causes minimal discomfort.

Acupuncture has been found to be effective in treating a variety of painful disorders, both acute and chronic. The World Health Organisation in 1979 drew up the following provisional list of disorders that lend themselves to acupuncture treatment. The list is based on clinical experience and not necessarily controlled clinical research:

1. Digestive disorders such as gastritis, hyperacidity, spastic bowl, constipation, and diarrhoea.
2. Respiratory disorders such as sinusitis, bronchitis, asthma.
3. Neurological and muscular disorders such as headaches, neck and back pain, neuralgia, frozen shoulder, tennis elbow, sciatica, and arthritis.
4. Urinary, menstrual, and reproductive disorders.
5. Addiction and substance abuse.
6. Sleep disorders such as insomnia and sleep apnea.

According to TCM, acupuncture works due to its effect on the essential substance that makes up the human body and enables it to sustain life activities and functions. This "substance," for a lack of a better word, is known as *Chi* or *Qi* (pronounced "chee").

Western biomedical research has learned that acupuncture works in certain situations by stimulating the body to produce endorphins, a morphine-like chemical that helps block pathways that relay pain messages. The result is relief from pain, general relaxation, and restoring the body's own internal regulatory system.

The Dao of Herbs

A primer on traditional Chinese herbal tonics. The Daoist arts put almost immeasurable emphasis on cultivating the "Three Treasures.

In the Orient, all philosophy, art and science are traditionally based on the fundamental realization that all things and all processes are interconnected. Oriental wise men and women long ago recognised the interconnectedness of the various parts of the body. The human body, mind and spirit are experienced as one complete whole, within themselves, with the environment and with the universe.

The notion of the unity of the body and psyche is fundamental to the Oriental healing arts. Changes in one's physical condition will result in changes in one's thinking and in one's intuitive and emotional processes. The mind likewise directly and indirectly influences gross and subtle changes in one's physical nature and in the actions we take. Virtually all aspects of health are rooted in the harmonious integration of the body and the psyche.

The Oriental health-maintenance and health-promotion arts, such as tonic herbalism, take full advantage of this oneness of body and psyche to help each person to grow to as full a state of health, well-being and spiritual awareness as the person is ready to achieve. The tonic herbs are used to bring about changes in one's physical condition; simultaneously, they are routinely used to influence the conscious and subconscious mind, the emotions and the human spirit.

No form of health care is complete unless it recognizes and utilizes this principle of the unity of physical and psychic energy. A Chinese tonic herbalist will never attempt to influence a change in just one aspect of a person's physical or psychic life In any case, such an attempt would be fruitless.

The goal of tonic herbalism is to help the tonic herbs user to establish a harmony of body, mind and spirit which can result in a new level of well-being, a new level of health and happiness that forms the foundation for a creative, successful life, as well as for true spiritual discovery, growth and, possibly, eventual mastery and enlightenment.

Essential Energy of Foods

Traditional Chinese Medicine classifies foods by their energetic values rather than their caloric or fat content. Here is a list of popular foods and their classification.

Cold

Banana, Watermelon, Bok Choi, Turnip, Celery, Cauliflower, Crab, Bean Sprouts, Asparagus, Eggplant, Cucumber, Grapefruit, Pineapple, Tangerine, Zucchini, Seaweed, Tofu

Cool

Pear, Peppermint, Green Tea, Oolong Tea, Bittergourd, Cooked Lettuce, Green Apple, Snow Pea, White Corn, Oranges, Cabbage, Soyabean Sprouts, Apples, Cooked Onion, Strawberries, Cheese, Cherries, Mushrooms

Warm

Rice, Noodles, Bread, Pork, Chicken, Turkey, Broccoli, Green Pepper, Green Beans, Egg Whites, Yellow Corn, Egg Yolk, Fish, Pepper, Ginger, Garlic, Cooked Tomato, Spinach, Black Tea, Nectarines, Milk

Hot

Nuts, Grilled Foods, Avocado, Lichee, Turtle, Chocolate, Cocoa, Raw Onions, Coffee, Lamb, Duck, Eggplant, Red Pepper, Venison, Deep Fried Foods

In the Chinese spiritual axis (Ling Shu Jing), it is said, "If no food is eaten for half a day, Qi is weakened, if no food is eaten for a whole day, Qi is depleted." This clearly emphasizes the importance of dietary discipline in a lifestyle that is designed to enhance personal experience of *Qi*.

Although much of modern research and discussion of ways to enhance our experience of *Qi* revolve around body mind breathing disciplines such as Qigong and Taijiquan, traditional Chinese medicine recognizes dietary discipline as equally fundamental in this respect.

Indeed, in the Spiritual Axis (Ling Shu Jing), it is said that "If no food is eaten for half a day, *Qi* is weakened, if no food is eaten for a whole day, *Qi* is depleted." This clearly emphasizes the importance of dietary discipline in a lifestyle that is designed to enhance personal experience of *Qi*.

Interestingly, traditional Chinese medicine maintains that human *Qi* originates with what literally means "*Qi* of grains." Thus Chinese medicine recognises grains—in particular, rice, but also all other grains—as the foundation of human vitality.

In fact, according to Chinese herbology, the taste of grains is generally sweet, and this flavor tonifies the Spleen and Stomach, which together are the organs responsible for transforming gu-*Qi* into zhen-*Qi*, true human vitality.

The traditional Chinese diet reflects this understanding of the importance of grains, above all other foods, for the maintenance of human well-being. The Chinese have for centuries made grains—in Chinese, *fan*—the mainstays of their diet, and all other foods, whether vegetable or animal, are used as mere condiments, or *sung*, to enhance one's enjoyment of grain foods.

The wisdom of this grain based diet style has recently been corroborated by the massive China Health Project, an ongoing study of current dietary patterns in China by staff from the Chinese Academy of Preventive Medicine, and Oxford and Cornell Universities. The study has found that the health and nutritional status of the people of China is generally superior to that of the people of Western industrialised nations. In particular, the incidence of heart disease, cancer, and other degenerative diseases—which from the standpoint of Chinese medicine are disorders of Blood and *Qi*—is far lower in China than in the United States.

Researchers are concluding that this is largely due to the predominance of grains and minimal consumption of animal foods in the traditional Chinese diet, because the people who live in urban areas of China and eat a non-traditional diet with more animal foods and less grains have degenerative diseases at rates approaching those of western industrialized nations.

According to Cornell researcher T. Colin Campbell, one of the leaders of this study, the evidence is compelling enough that the World Health Organisation has asked him to co-author a document addressed to developing nations titled "More Meat Does Not Mean Better Health", and the government of China is putting a hold on its previous plans to develop a large livestock and dairy food industry.

Thus, modern nutritional epidemiology lends its support to the view of traditional Chinese medicine that grains are the essential source of humanity's *Qi*, health, vitality and longevity.

20
Practitioners

Naturopathy is profession that specialises in natural medicine. It blends old non-toxic therapies with a current understanding of health and human systems.

Naturopaths practise comprehensive medical care and treat the whole person. It recognises the body's inherent healing abilities. And it identifies the underlying causes of disease rather than suppresses symptoms. It prevents disease through promoting a healthy lifestyle and educating the patient. But asking someone to change what they eat is the hardest thing in the world to do.

Herbal medicine and homeopathy, manipulation are a big part of naturopathy. Naturopaths do adjustments on the entire body, not just the spine. We also do hydrotherapy and hypnosis.

Naturopathy has its origins in the Nature Cure movement of Europe. The term was coined in 1895 by John Scheel and popularised by Benedict Lust, the "father of U.S. naturopathy".

Naturopathy is practised in many countries, and is subject to different standards of regulation and levels of acceptance. The level of medical education among naturopaths also varies, though no naturopathic training programmme reaches the same level of training as an MD or DO.

The scope of practice varies widely between jurisdictions, and naturopaths in unregulated jurisdictions may use the

Naturopathic Doctor designation or other titles regardless of level of education.

Naturopathy does not offer a magic cure, although many report very rapid results. Truly great results come from positive behavior changes and the persistence it requires to maintain these changes long enough for the body to respond.

The Naturopathic physician is trying to stimulate and support the patient's own system to address the imbalance(s) that have damaged their health. Often, long-term underlying disturbances such as nutritional deficiencies or excesses, rather than the presenting health problem, must be corrected in order to allow the body to reassert its natural state of optimal health. Our elders called these "Impediments to Cure."

The cornerstones of Naturopathic philosophy are prevention and responsibility for one's own health. Naturopathic treatments often are based on assessing risk factors connected to the patient's lifestyle, diet, and environment. Each of these factors is taken under consideration when developing a treatment plan with a client. The goal is to remove obstacles to the patient's own state of optimal health.

Once the patient's history has been taken, the Naturopath may do a screening physical, which is a standard physical examination supplemented by in-depth questions, and may seek laboratory testing or diagnostic imaging of the complaint. After the intake and physical are completed, the Naturopath will discuss the treatment plan or protocol with the patient.

If needed, the patient will be referred for laboratory or other diagnostic tests, or to their medical doctor for further consultation. Follow-up visits are scheduled from one to four weeks after treatment has begun. If a chronic illness is being addressed, the patient can expect to undergo at least one month of treatment for every year of illness.

In brief, homeopaths use only the homoeopathic approach, whereas Naturopaths train in several forms of diagnosis and treatment, one of which is homeopathy. Training in homeopathy varies from a several-hundred-hour correspondence course to a three/four-year course for which candidates need not be university graduates. In contrast, Naturopaths must complete a minimum of three years of university training prior to beginning their four-year residential medical school training in Naturopathic Medicine.

Naturopathic physicians are primary health care practitioners. They are trained to be the doctor who is first seen by the patient for general health care, advice on keeping healthy, and the diagnosis and treatment of acute and chronic conditions.

For treatment it primarily stresses on correcting all the factors involved and allowing the body to recover itself. A Nature Cure physician helps in Nature's effort to overcome disease by applying correct natural modalities and controlling the natural forces to work within safe limits. The five main modalities of treatment are air, water, heat, mud and space.

They also serve those whose treatment by conventional means has not met their needs and who seek naturopathic care as an alternative.

Naturopathic medical degrees are referred to both as NMD or ND. The current scope of naturopathic practice includes, but is not limited to:

1. Clinical Nutrition
2. Botanical Medicine
3. Homoeopathic Medicine
4. Physical Medicine
5. Oriental Medicine
6. Naturopathic Obstetrics
7. Psychological Medicine
8. Minor Surgery

Naturopathy Courses

Continuing education in naturopathic modalities for health care professionals varies greatly but includes offerings for many professions, including physicians, physical therapists, chiropractors, acupuncturists, dentists, researchers, veterinarians, physician assistants, and nurses. These professionals usually retain their original designation but may use terms such as 'holistic', 'natural', or 'integrative' to describe their practice.

In India there is a 5 1/2 year degree course offering a Bachelor of Naturopathy and Yogic Sciences (BNYS) degree. There are a total of 11 colleges in India, of which 4 colleges are in the state of Tamil Nadu.

Naturopathic practice does not include the primary use of most synthetic drugs and major surgery, although naturopathic physicians refer patients to specialists if these are indicated.

Naturopathic physicians are well-trained in all modern methods of diagnostic testing, including X-ray, ultrasound, and other imaging techniques.

The majority of naturopathic physicians are in general, private practice. Some, however, choose to emphasize particular treatment modalities, some of which are listed above. Or they may concentrate in particular medical fields such as pediatrics, gynecology, allergies, arthritis, etc.

It is important to distinguish licensed naturopathic physicians from non-licensed practitioners who have completed only short-term course work, mostly by correspondence.

Naturopathic Doctors

Naturopathy is a holistic system, meaning that naturopathic doctors (NDs) or naturopathic medical doctors (NMDs) strive to find the cause of disease by understanding the patient as a totality of body, mind, and spirit. Most naturopathic doctors use a wide variety of therapies and techniques (such as nutrition, herbal medicine, homeopathy, and acupuncture).

Modern naturopathic physicians (NDs) use therapies that are primarily natural and non-toxic. These include clinical nutrition, homeopathy, botanical medicine, hydrotherapy, physical medicine, and counseling. Many NDs have additional training and certification in acupuncture and home birthing. These contemporary NDs, who have attended naturopathic medical colleges, practice medicine as primary health care providers and are increasingly acknowledged as leaders of change in the medical system,

Today's naturopathic physicians continue to use these therapies as their main tools and advocate a healthy dose of primary prevention. In addition, modern NDs conduct and make practical use of the latest bio-chemical research involving nutrition, botanicals, homeopathy, and other natural treatments. For many diseases and conditions (a few examples are ulcerative colitis, asthma, meno-pause, flu, obesity, and chronic fatigue), treatments used by naturopathic physicians can be primary and even curative.

Naturopathic physicians also function within an integrated framework, partnering with practitioners of conventional medicine. Naturopathic therapies can also be employed to complement treatments used by conventionally trained doctors. The result is a team-care approach that recognizes the needs of the patient to receive the best overall treatment most appropriate to his or her specific medical condition.

Future Prospects

In a few years, Naturopathy has made great progress. In the developing world, where traditional knowledge still survives, Naturopathy has always been widely used. The first years of a new millennium, as we look out towards a better, more mature, and wiser world, where the oneness of all things is beginning to be understood, Naturopathy will reinforce long forgotten links with Mother Earth on one hand, whilst fostering a healthier world on the other.

What do Naturopathic Doctors do?

Naturopathic doctors do not undergo the same training as medical doctors do. For example, they are not required to complete residency training.

In training, there may be less emphasis on clinical science and they may be educated in areas like homeopathy and vitalism, which contradict or stand in opposition to conventional medical treatments; for example, naturopathic doctors may suggest the use of vitamins, mineral supplements and other natural materials instead of prescription drugs. However, at the end of their training, they can be board-certified and practice as primary care providers.

Those interested in seeing a naturopath should be aware that traditional naturopaths don't undergo as much official training as board-certified naturopathic doctors.

Regardless of the efficacy and varied definitions of any naturopathic medicine methods, many practitioners attempt to adhere to an ideology that uses naturally-occurring and non-invasive methods that are guided by six core values, which exist in different forms, but include: doing no harm, respecting the self-healing power of the body, identifying and removing the causes of illness, encourage the patient's responsibility for his health, consider all health factors unique to an individual, and the emphasize the benefit of good health in preventing disease in individuals and entire communities.

With the guiding principle of relatively harmless, non-invasive treatment, many naturopathic medicine practices depend on eliminating and preventing disease with methods that do not treat ailments directly, but though holistic or indirect approaches.

Proponents believe that naturopathic medicine, by treating causes and not symptoms, leads to better overall health by preventing future recurrence of the ailment.

Some naturopathic methods have become accepted by many medical doctors and some jurisdictions have practice guidelines for MDs to incorporate naturopathic medicine in their practice.

❖❖❖

21

Philosophy

Living things have an innate ability to heal themselves. Our vital force promotes self-cleansing, self-repair, and therefore self-healing. This process can be achieved by focusing on the immune, hormonal, nervous, and detoxification/elimination systems of the body. Once these systems are in balance, restored health is a probability.

The body possesses the power to heal itself through its internal vitality. This vital force is the foundation of naturopathic philosophy. All that the naturopathic practitioner does is to create the most favourable condition to stimulate and enhance natural healing power.

Modern life all over the world has taken its own toll on man. Environmental degradation has assumed alarming proportions. One has heard repeated warnings of global warming and depletion of the ozone layer in recent times. The WHO has pinpointed rapid rise in pollution levels the world over as being the single largest cause of cardiovascular disease, much more than smoking. Moreover, adulterated food and use of highly toxic pesticides that destroy the nutritive value of foodgrains and vegetables have taken a toll too.

Moreover, modern man leads a much more sedentary lifestyle than his ancestors did. He has reached the "Remote control" stage of technological progress. It is not surprising at all that he should find it imperative to regulate his diet and work out at the gym. Add to that the stresses and strains of the modern consumerist world, and man is not exactly happier than what he used to be.

Medical science itself seems to have reached a plateau now, and has got bogged down by the ethical implications of anything between donating sperm to cloning human beings. Besides, despite all the advancement, age-old maladies such as diabetes and asthma are far from curable. They are at best controllable. Most antibiotics seem inadequate in tackling viral infections. Bacteria that cause other diseases have developed resistance to certain types of antibiotics. Besides, the common man himself has become somewhat wary of allopathic medicines and has begun to turn to alternative, traditional forms of medicine.

This has in recent times brought about a welcome change in attitudes that were hitherto prevalent in the medical world. Much prejudice against alternative systems of medicine seems to have been shed and a They are no more the fanciful fad of the famous or the poor substitute of the underprivileged. They are now being increasingly acknowledged as viable, alternative systems of healing the sick.

Disease is a manifestation of the vital force applying itself to the removal of obstruction to the normal functioning of organs and tissues.

Naturopathic treatments originated as the use of herbs and foods for medicine, exposure to fresh air and sunlight, and hydrotherapy (the use of hot and cold water application) as steam or sauna. These techniques and methods have long been respected throughout the world.

While modern allopathic medicine is a youngster of less than 200 years old, Natural Medicine has been the primary medicine used by most of the human community even into the 21st Century. Herbal and traditional medical arts remain the primary medical choice of over 65 per cent of humanity.

A growing public interest in alternative or complementary medicine to maintain and restore health has led to a resurgence of belief in the importance of diet, lifestyle, personal choice to ideal health. This validated the original principles and teachings of the naturopathic profession.

Naturopathic medicine in practice considers the fundamental components of health - biochemistry, biomechanics, and the emotional predisposition - in order to help a person restore the balance that we describe as good health. This philosophy empowers the individual as being responsible for the level of health they experience.

Naturopathic medicine offers safe, cost-effective solutions for many of our nation's healthcare problems. Competence and respect for tradition, the scientific method, and innovation are hallmarks of a naturopathic medical practice.

Naturopathic doctors treat their patients holistically, taking into consideration the individual's biochemistry, biomechanics, and emotional predispositions. The body's self-healing ability can be better understood if one takes into account the fact that homeostasis, or biological balance, is the main characteristic of any healthy system.

A good example is fever. When the body is invaded by a pathogen (a substance capable of producing illness or disease), the body will usually respond by producing a fever to fight the invader. If the body is properly supported through nutrition and rest, the fever will turn up the immune system and permit the recovery of health.

Other examples are the immune system, hormonal system, nervous system, and detoxification/elimination pathways, which all work as a unit to ensure our survival. If given the proper support, care, and the chance to function freely without suppression, they can bring the system back to a state of balance or "ease" (as opposed to "dis-ease").

There are no panaceas or magic bullets. Each individual has his or her own unique set of symptoms and reactions which will, in turn, dictate the approach the naturopathic doctor takes to treat them. This is why each person seeking help from a naturopathic doctor will receive an individualised treatment protocol. Naturopathic medicine is practiced either as a primary system of medical care, or as a complementary adjunct to conventional medical treatment.

The goal of naturopathic medicine is to develop optimal wellness for each patient, and to teach the principles of ideal health. Although Naturopathic doctors are educated and trained to treat acute and chronic disease, prevention is the ultimate goal. This is based on the naturopathic philosophy of wellness enhancement — not disease management.

The naturopathic axiom that "nature-cures" is largely forgotten in the world of modern medicine. We have become accustomed to modern drug therapy that overrides the understanding and realisation of our body's own healing power. Without this innate healing power we would remain in the disease state.

Perhaps the body is ever in a disease state but for the continual actuation of the unconscious healing mechanisms, we keep ourselves in a balanced state we term health. The naturopath sees the patient in the context of health, and not from what disease he or she may be experiencing. This subtle approach is radically different to modern medicine. The naturopath does not treat symptoms but uses these to indicate how the self-healing power is attempting to rectify the inner state of disharmony. For example, fever is a natural rising of the body's temperature to achieve a cleansing of the blood of toxins and metabolic wastes. It is not something to be suppressed but carefully encouraged to achieve its aim.

The naturopath is one who observes and uses Nature's laws in obtaining a balance or harmony within the individual. This wisdom has been handed down through the ages in traditional medicine and folk remedies. This has largely been put aside in the belief that modern science knows better than the secrets of the forces or wisdom of Nature. The naturopath reasserts traditional wisdom in light of modern understanding.

By and large, the modern diseases arise from our abnormal social living and not according to Nature's laws. The degradation of food quality, increased environment toxicity and the preponderance of stressful and one-sided living, leads to the condition of nutrient deficiency and body toxicity.

Rectify deficiency and toxicity, medicine of any kind, be it natural or chemical are only secondary.

The Hippocratic adage of "Let food be your medicine and medicine be your food" becomes central to establishing inner harmony. We experience health when the channels of elimination are open; these are the bowels, liver, kidneys, lungs and skin. Toxicity invariably occurs when these channels are blocked or stagnant. The most challenging of disease states can be successfully treated with nutrition and detoxification. Chemical drugs only exacerbate the toxicity of the body - this is why the naturopath only uses natural medicine and techniques.

Naturopathy is holistic medicine and recognises the spirit in man. The soul is our essence and the expression of Divinity. The naturopath addresses the soul of the patient in the totality of the life he or she leads. A patient's emotional outlook is a key to the maintenance of health and a bearing on the recovery of health.

❖❖❖